Prostate Cancer Treatment Options

A Guide To The Basics

by

Will Connell

With Forewords by

Ross Z. Pierpont, M.D.
President, CEO, Pierpont Systems
Consultants International,
and formerly Chief of Surgery,
Maryland General Hospital

Mack Roach III, M.D.
Associate Professor of Radiation Oncology,
Medical Oncology and Urology,
University of California, San Francisco, California

Charles K. Metzger, M.D.
Urologic Surgeon, Glendora, California

John Kurhanewicz, Ph.D.
Assistant Professor of Radiology,
Magnetic Resonance Science Center,
University of California, San Francisco, California

Edconco Press
Grass Valley, California

Prostate Cancer Treatment Options

A Guide to the Basics

Published by Edconco Press
PO Box 357
Grass Valley, California 95945
U.S.A.

SAN:299-9676
Printed in Hong Kong

Internet Site: www.prostatecanceroptions.com

Library of Congress Catalog Card Number: 99-95100
Publisher's Cataloging-in-Publication
(Provided by Quality Books, Inc.)
Connell, Will, 1935-
Prostate cancer treatment options : a guide to
the basics / Will Connell.—1st ed.
p. cm.
Includes bibliographical references and index.
ISBN: 0-9673892-1-6

1. Prostate—Cancer—Popular works.
I. Title.

RC280.P7C66 1999 616.99'463
QBI99 -1253

Cover and color graphics by Ken Sheffer, Omega Group
Typography and text layout by Jill Cremer, Visions Design Services,
and George Van Buren of Van Buren Designs
Editing by Saundra Sheffer and Judie Rae

Disclaimer

This guide is intended only as a source of information for the reader who is planning his prostate cancer therapy in consultation with a health care provider.

The reader is warned that this guide should not be the basis for any decision without consideration of its contents with his health care provider. The author cannot be liable for actions that may be taken by the reader as a result of information contained in this guide. Patients, working in concert with a licensed physician, are responsible for their ultimate treatment decisions.

The author advises the patient to consult with a number of physicians before embarking upon any treatment program for prostate cancer.

The author does not endorse or oppose any treatment mentioned in this guide. He is not a medical authority, so his ideas and suggestions ought to be read with this fact in mind. He has collected information from a number of sources deemed reliable, including published books and articles from newspapers and medical journals. The guide is sold with the understanding that neither the author nor the publisher is associated in any way with the medical profession nor in any aspect of medical counseling.

The author and publisher acknowledge that errors, both typographical and with regard to content, either included or excluded, are inherent in the text. Treatment of prostate cancer is a fast-moving medical field, and data on this subject change daily. Much relevant information has been excluded from the guide as an expediency for the reader. This guide is presented only as a general educational device for the patient. The statistical information contained in the guide must be verified by your physician if you are to make decisions based upon it.

It is agreed and understood that you accept the foregoing disclaimer. If you do not wish to be bound by the above, you may return this book to the publisher within two weeks, for a full refund.

Some of the funds generated by this publication will be donated to charitable organizations involved with cancer research.

Contents

Acknowledgements

I wish to thank my wife, Judie, my daughter, Eve, my sister and brother-in-law, Samantha and Arch MacPhail, my friends Saundra and Ken Sheffer, Robert Edwards, Mark Liggett, Malcolm Seagrave, Myrna and George Van Buren, Ed Forys, Art Gottlieb, Dr. George and Mrs. Jean Kidera, Dr. Jared Spotkov, Dr. David Underwood, and my physicians, Dr. Stuart Fisher, Dr. Jeffrey Frost, Dr. John Kurhanewicz, Dr. Charles Metzger, Dr. Mack Roach, Dr. Katsuto Shinohara, and Dr. Eric Vigneault, all of whom supported me and guided me through an incredible adventure, one that has turned out to be a surprisingly rewarding and truly life-enhancing experience.

Will Connell
Grass Valley
California
2000

Foreword

This book is a well thought out, clearly written, exhaustive study of the nature of prostate cancer, its diagnosis and available treatment.

The book can be a realistic help to any man and his family faced with decisions of what to do in the case of diagnosed cancer of the prostate.

The short chapters, and the summaries closing each chapter, enhance the ability to understand the material presented.

Overall, this is a helpful book and recommended for purchase by individuals faced with the problem of prostate cancer.

Ross Z. Pierpont, M.D., F.A.C.S.
President, CEO
Pierpont Systems Consultants International
Timonium, Maryland
Formerly Chief of Surgery
Maryland General Hospital

Foreword

The average patient usually presents for treatment in a daze about what is happening to him. He most likely has not read much literature on the subject and thus is not in an optimistic frame of mind. I believe the approach in this guide could play a critical role in the decision-making process for many patients.

This approach to solving the education problem is a powerful one. It is reader-friendly. This work introduces the patient to the basics so that he can make an educated decision about treatment. The author is wise in not presenting all the fine details, many of which are debated in the medical professions. Such details only serve to deter the new patient from learning the essentials and developing a positive attitude.

I think this work will go a long way in relieving the suffering that so many men face. With nearly 200,000 new prostate cancer cases being diagnosed each year, this book is greatly needed.

Mack Roach III, M.D.
Associate Professor of Radiation Oncology
Medical Oncology and Urology
University of California
San Francisco, California

Foreword

At last, a book written by a patient with a scientific approach making critical prostate cancer treatment decisions. I am a urologic surgeon and have always favored surgical treatment. However, new advances in diagnosis, staging, and treatment of prostate cancer have changed this straightforward recommendation. The newly diagnosed patient with localized disease has many more options to consider for primary treatment.

Utilizing his aerospace training the author has worked out decision flow charts that helped him, and they can definitely help others in the decision process. This is an extraordinary approach that will benefit anyone who is faced with these cancer-related decisions.

This book lays out the basic considerations that any man faces with his diagnosis of prostate cancer. New radiation techniques, alternate therapies, hormone treatment, and standard surgical treatments are all discussed rationally. The extraneous information often found in traditional medicine is kept in perspective as well as is the pervasive "fee for service mentality" that often clouds the decision-making process.

I highly recommend this book to any newly diagnosed prostate cancer patient

Charles K. Metzger, M.D., M.B.A.
Citrus Valley Urologic Medical Group, Inc.
Glendora, California

Foreword

Because of prostate cancer screening using serum prostate-specific antigen (PSA) and transrectal prostate ultrasound guided biopsy, thousands of prostate cancer patients like Will Connell are being identified at an earlier and potentially treatable stage. However, the decision on how to manage prostate cancer once it is diagnosed poses a great dilemma for both patients and their doctors. The dilemma stems from the fact that prostate cancers demonstrate a tremendous range in biologic malignancy and are treated with a broad spectrum of approaches from "watchful waiting" and hormone ablation therapy to aggressive surgical, radiation, and cryosurgical therapies. As some prostate cancer patients already know there is no one "right" answer for everyone, and the decision as to whether and how to treat their cancer becomes a personal decision. Mr. Connell and I both believe that it is important for any new patient to learn as much as possible so he can take command of his situation. This guide introduces the patient to the basics of prostate cancer using everyday terms so that the patient can make an educated decision.

Unfortunately, the information available on prostate cancer can still be overwhelming, and the differences in opinion concerning its treatment are disconcerting for the average patient. Connell, being both a prostate cancer survivor and a scientist, has been able to bring into focus all the important aspects of prostate cancer faced by a newly diagnosed patient. Visually he shows the new patient what features of his unique medical condition to consider, so that he will not be side-tracked by overwhelming information that could lead to frustration and despair.

This guide also stresses just how important accurate imaging is in therapeutic selection and planning. Recent improvements in magnetic resonance imaging technology and the addition of functional or metabolic information (magnetic resonance spectroscopic imaging - MRSI) have allowed a more accurate assessment of the location, spatial extent and aggressiveness of a tumor than was previously possible. Confidence in the decision-making process can be greatly increased by combining this imaging information with other clinical parameters.

I believe this guide will serve the new patient well as he plots his own course to a successful treatment outcome.

John Kurhanewicz, Ph.D.
Assistant Professor of Radiology
Magnetic Resonance Science Center
University of California
San Francisco, California

Introduction

If you have been recently diagnosed with prostate cancer, you are not alone. This year about 200,000 men received this news. Prostate cancer is the most commonly discovered cancer in men, after skin cancers; one out of every ten men will be diagnosed during their lives. It is the second leading cause of cancer death in men, after lung cancer. About one man in 200 will die from this cause. These are frightening statistics, but the good news is that because of earlier detection and improved medical techniques, the number of men who will die because of prostate cancer is being drastically reduced.

Almost 60% of new cases are discovered while the tumor is still confined within the prostate, so the five-year survival rate for men with localized prostate cancer is 100%. Some 30% of men are discovered with tumor material that has escaped the prostate, so the survival rate drops to about 94%. Even with the 10% of men newly diagnosed with cancer that has already spread to distant parts of the body, the five-year survival rate is about 30%, and there are many new techniques that will improve even this statistic.

This guide is intended to offer any man a method to manage the dilemma he faces upon hearing that he has prostate cancer. You will hear many opinions, obtain many physicians' diagnoses, study books, learn true and untrue aspects of this prevalent condition. (Note that I refer to this as a condition, not a disease, as it is commonly represented to be. You will soon learn why I think this.)

I also hope to reach the reader who does not have prostate cancer, or who may be a young man. This guide will outline what may lie before you, and subsequent chapters will discuss dietary factors that many believe influence prostate cancer initiation and growth. In retrospect, as a young man I would have benefited from the knowledge outlined in this guide.

Finally, you will wish to know what new technologies are on the horizon, and there are chapters giving brief reviews of these exciting developments.

Chapter 1

Why This Guide?

I suppose that every person who successfully surmounts a potentially life-threatening dilemma has an urge to tell others about it and share what he has learned, even perhaps by writing a book. One does not confront the real possibility of death and continue to regard life the same as before. I have succumbed to the temptation to write a book, but not because I think my situation is in any way unique. On the contrary, my research has shown me how common prostate cancer is. I want to share my insights and experience with others who may be facing the same situation.

You may be interested in the subject because a loved one has the condition, or because you have been diagnosed with prostate cancer yourself. I faced the same fears you may have and was forced to make decisions that would affect the rest of my life. I think my *approach* to this decision-making process is unique, especially when I compare it to the publications I have come across.

Not everyone has the time or the wherewithal to visit a number of clinics and conduct his own research regarding the optimum treatment solution to his condition. Many books on the subject give the reader *too much* information. Talking to men during my therapy taught me that these books can be counter-productive, because some overwhelmed readers give up in despair, believing that they could never absorb all the information that is presented to them. Such books often are put aside before the reader has a chance to absorb even the basics. That is why I am setting down my experience and research in this guide. I hope that my approach makes clear just the bare treatment basics and what you need to know for a proper treatment decision. I want to demystify the issues, so you can plot your course to the successful treatment of *your* particular cancer condition. I have tried hard to present my conclusions in a simple and visual way.

You may be confused at first as to where to turn, what to do, and how to sort through conflicting information. This book is a guide, not a comprehensive explanation of prostate cancer. It tells you only the basics of what you need to know and suggests ways to evaluate the treatment that may be appropriate for you. You will be able to determine where *you* are in the scheme of things and forget about the other aspects of prostate cancer. This guide should relieve your anxiety by showing you that most likely you are not in immediate danger because of prostate cancer.

My background is in science, but as much as I studied, I was unable to find what I needed to visualize the treatment choices appropriate for *my* particular situation, so I went further in my research. I read scientific papers in professional cancer and urology journals, and I thought hard about the issues that I faced. Only then was I able to construct decision-making guidelines that included all the trade-offs — the benefits, the risks, the advantages, and disadvantages — that I could discuss with my physicians.

My research and personal experiences resulted in the Treatment Option Charts and Future Treatment Options Chart presented in Chapter 9.

You face a dilemma: What is the most effective way to treat *your* particular cancer condition? What are the side effects and quality of life issues that accompany a particular treatment and will affect the rest of *your* life? The Future Treatment Options Chart clarifies this critical dilemma, and should help you decide on your primary therapy.

This guide focuses on how you can arrive at an orderly and sensible approach to your particular dilemma, perhaps using my guides as a starting point for your journey, a journey that you should take with your physician as a *partner*.

I was surprised to learn how many men take a fatalistic approach to prostate cancer. During my treatments, I heard men say things like: "These are the cards that were dealt me and the doctors will do the best as they can." Or, "I only hope that I have found a good doctor to treat me." I believe that a positive approach will assist the doctors and result in your achieving a far better outcome than that of the patient who is passive or blindly submits to authority.

The path to the best solution can be so confusing that you may be tempted to throw up your hands and let a comforting and/or decisive physician do the decision-making for you. I believe that if we do that we lessen our chances for complete recovery, perhaps endangering ourselves in the process. When you choose not to engage yourself fully in the decision-making process, your attitude changes from a positive "take-charge" attitude to a passive, negative one. If you take command of your own destiny and face your physician almost as an equal, your chances are greatly improved.

Prostate cancer, as we know, is finally gaining wider public awareness. It is no longer a forbidden topic for discussion. Perhaps because this condition strikes at the very core of our masculinity it has not been a subject of widespread media attention or public discussion. Only in the past two or three years has public consciousness been raised. We are only now learning that cancer may be a built-in part of the multicellular life of higher animals. Almost all men, if they live long enough, will develop prostate cancer. It is not to be thought of as a disease that one contracts. Prostate cancer is a *condition* that comes with aging and being male.The following table will make this point:

Age	Cancer Rate
40 – 60	30% have signs of pre-cancer or incipient cancer
60 – 70	30% have active tumor present
70 – 80	40% have active tumor present
80 – 90	80% have active tumor present
90 +	Approaches 100%

Table 1
Prostate Cancer and Aging

One has to conclude from these numbers that prostate cancer is a condition of life, not merely a disease that strikes some and not others. Indeed, autopsies performed on men of all ages tend to support the idea that as we age we all generate what are called microfoci or tiny "latent" prostate cancers. The incidence of these tiny cancers appears to increase with age. These investigations show that 30 percent of men over age 50 are thus afflicted. About half of all prostate cancer patients are first diagnosed between ages 60 and 70, and two-thirds of them report no symptoms before the discovery. It appears that if we live long enough, almost all of us will develop prostate cancer. It has been said that most men will die, not of the cancer itself, but with the cancer, when other causes of death finally appear. One may conclude that those who reach extreme age without producing prostate cancer are the exception, not those of us who develop cancer along the way.

Until recently we did not know the true extent of this condition. It is only through the use of new blood testing, a greater awareness of health matters in general, increased longevity, improved studies of environment and the role of carcinogens, and more regular physical examinations, that accurate statistical data have been obtained. This leads many doctors to urge men over age fifty to have a regular prostate specific antigen test to determine his own PSA level, perhaps annually or every other year.

This is particularly advisable if prostate cancer has occurred in your father, brother, or uncle. A history of prostate cancer within your family is *your* most important risk factor. If one man in your family has the condition, your risk is twice the normal risk. If two family members have the condition, your risk is four to six times the norm. Johns Hopkins researchers report that if a family has a dominant gene for prostate cancer, the risk of developing this cancer by age 85 approaches 100 percent.

African-American men have a 32 percent higher rate of

prostate cancer than do white American men, and they are twice as likely to develop this condition while they are still in their early fifties.

When very young men are diagnosed with prostate cancer, their tumors seem to be more aggressive than normal. Curiously, such patients also show cancer developing at PSA levels lower than what would be considered a dangerous level for their age bracket.

With society's growing awareness of prostate cancer, cancer screening tests will become routine for all men. When this happens there will be no reason for any man to develop advanced cancer; hence, no man ought to die of this condition. In early 1998 an eight-year Canadian study showed that medical screening can reduce deaths by 69 percent. More than 27,000 lives could be saved annually by such screenings, the report said.

As you age and receive the results from your annual medical reviews, your physician will be watching a number of factors relating to your potential for developing prostate cancer. Figure 1 (see center section containing color charts) is a visual summary of many risk factors. You may wish to locate where you are in these risk categories.

Remember This

All men face the prospect of prostate cancer. If you have loved ones, you have obligations and responsibilities. If you are a young man, you have goals for the future. Your first responsibility must be your own health. You, and only you, are responsible for your health. If you fail this basic responsibility, you will fail all the others.

This guide is oriented toward treatment decision-making. It outlines a method that you can use to determine an appropriate solution to your treatment dilemma. Some of the things shown here may be at odds with the published

literature available to the layman. They may be different from what you are told by your physician. Some of the ideas may be controversial enough to antagonize members of the medical profession.

Prostate cancer treatment is a rapidly evolving field and what was last year's standard practice, could be outdated next year. If we could look ten years ahead we might be amazed at the advances in treatments, as well as the changes in attitude about treatment procedure. Many of today's therapies will be completely outmoded.

My conclusions come as a result of my successful treatment experience, two years of research, many consultations with physicians working at the cutting edge of these new technologies, and the application of a bit of common sense.

When people are hurt or scared they may do desperate things. This guide outlines the things I learned and used to make my decision. If you read something here that seems, at first, to be controversial to you, take a moment to reflect, study further, and discuss it with your physician. It may be something completely new, or may already be outdated, especially if you are reading this guide several years after its publication date.

Please remember that your life has value and worth. That is why I have written this guide.

Chapter 2

To Begin

So you have the news. You have this dreaded cancer. What are you going to do?

You are alarmed, angry, perhaps frightened. "It's not fair!" "I've never done anything to deserve this!" "I've been taking my zinc all these years, haven't I?" "After three decades of hard work, just when everything was starting to go my way at last, this has to happen." "How could this be happening to me?"

Your feelings may run the gamut from panic: "Cut that damned thing out as soon as possible," to denial. And on top of these strong feelings is confusion. You will be confused when you try to sort out not only your emotions regarding the news, but what to believe and what course to follow.

All of these reactions are normal and valid. It is important for you to have them. It will be helpful to work through them, sharing them with family, friends, support groups, and your doctor.

After you recover from the initial shock...fight back! Don't just sit there feeling sorry for yourself. Attack! In doing so you will find that you will feel much better about yourself, and your chances of survival will increase, too. Neither panic nor denial helps you reach a proper solution to your condition. Once you realize this, you can take a reasoned approach to what to do next. There are a number of basic things you need to know, and by learning them you will gain the self-confidence you need to master the situation. The first thing you need to know is this:

Surgeons tend to recommend surgery.
Radiologists tend to recommend radiation.
Cryosurgeons tend to recommend freezing.
Dietary specialists will recommend diet cures.
Preachers will recommend faith.

"When your tool is a hammer, every problem resembles

a nail," and doctors, preachers, or dietary experts see problems and solutions from the perspective of their specialties. This comment may seem a bit harsh. There are truths in each of these treatment options. And there are pitfalls, some of which could lead to very unhappy consequences for you. This is the dilemma before you.

It is up to you to learn the basic facts about your cancer and to study each of the approaches to treatment. You should realize that by the time the tumor has been discovered by your physician, it has been there for some time, most likely for years. You can be as calm as possible as you go about your education and treatment choice decision. You probably do not have to take decisive action by next Wednesday. You have some time to approach your condition with deliberation and growing confidence. Figure 2 , taken from the book by Marks, shows the growth of tumors over time. Unless you have obvious physical symptoms, such as pain, your cancer most likely has been discovered while you are still in the "window of opportunity."

You must realize two important things:

1. *You* can be in control of your own destiny. You must not merely follow anyone who advocates only *one* of the possibilities. (In fact, an honorable physician will recommend that you investigate competing treatment methods. Whether or not he does this can serve as a test of the integrity of your present physician).

I recommend that second and third opinions be sought from *oncologists* who specialize in prostate cancer. I have met many prostate cancer survivors who are unhappy with the choice of treatment they made. They often say, "If I had to do it over again, I would have done more research." I decided that I would not allow myself to receive treatment of *any* kind without knowing about the full range of treatment possibilities available to me and of the potential side effects associated with each treatment. I felt that I should deal only with specialists in the prostate cancer field.

You should learn about the full range of treatment options available to you. In fact, you should be able to relate to each of your physicians almost on an equal footing, filled with as much knowledge as he has regarding the possibilities before you. Remember that each physician believes that his particular approach offers the most satisfactory method for resolving your situation. He believes his own abilities offer the best care that can be obtained by you. He may be right, but you must not assume that he knows the complete range of alternate possibilities or the downside consequences of each of them.

When you present yourself for treatment you will want to be in the best possible frame of mind. With confidence, you will be far more relaxed, and this will immeasurably help you rid yourself of cancer.

2. *You* should decide what to do and what course to follow. Your physician cannot know your internal emotions, your particular fears or desires, or your priorities in life. All this is happening to *you*, and this fact separates you from your doctors. In order to decide calmly and sensibly, you should take control of your emotions as soon as possible. This requires discipline, study, and time. With proper research, you will be able to confront the situation rationally, calmly, and confidently.

I do not endorse any particular procedure I write about in this book, nor do I reject any procedure mentioned in this book. This guide will chronicle *my* treatment choice analysis, a procedure that gave me confidence every step of the way to *my* successful treatment for prostate cancer.

Perhaps it will assist you in your journey.

Remember This

One of the surprising, perhaps noble, aspects of human

nature is that during times of stress, when confronting a major crisis, we discover hidden reserves of strength within ourselves. If you have been diagnosed with prostate cancer it is important to give yourself time to tap this reserve.

Unless you are diagnosed with an aggressive tumor or an advanced stage condition, you do not need to hurry your decision process. The medical profession tells us that the wisest course is to have a confident, fully educated patient rather than one who is uneducated and frightened. It is far more important for you to spend the time necessary to educate yourself to arrive at the optimum treatment decision, than it is to take quick action to treat your condition.

This guide should help prepare you fully, so you will present yourself for treatment as a patient who has tapped his hidden resource of strength.

Chapter 3

What Is Prostate Cancer?

This guide will not go into great detail about what prostate cancer is. However, there are a few basic things you need to know. We read more and more frequently that there is an "epidemic" of prostate cancer, that it is becoming more prevalent and is being identified more often than in the past.

The first thing you need to realize is that it is not a communicable disease as the word "epidemic" might imply. Prostate cancer cannot be contracted the way one might catch the flu or HIV. The underlying cause of cancer is not known with certainty. Most likely prostate cancer develops as a result of age, heredity, injury, diet, or exposure to carcinogens in our environment. It may be that a combination of these factors, operating over a period of years, is necessary for cancer to begin.

Thus, we can regard prostate cancer more as a condition that develops as we age. I suppose that what the sensationalist news items really mean by the word "epidemic" is that the medical community is becoming more and more familiar with the condition because new developments in testing are detecting it far earlier and more frequently than in the past. The old digital rectal exams are being complemented by sophisticated blood testing, sonogram imaging, and simplified biopsy sampling.

If it is not a disease, what is prostate cancer? It appears that prostate cancer is a group of cells that attempts to mimic the host tissue, the prostate gland. Tumor cells appear to develop in reaction to some chemical or genetic insult or injury of some kind to the normal prostate tissue. Or perhaps some men suffer from a genetic inheritance for certain cancers. Scientists don't know for sure what factors promote cancer growth.

In the late 19th century, Dr. Rudolph Virchow of Germany was famous for his discoveries in cellular pathology. His statement that "all cells come from other cells" changed medicine forever. It follows, then, that there are as many varieties of cancer as there are organs and tissues within the body. By identifying the cell as the ultimate unit of life and disease, Virchow paved the way for chemotherapy in this century.

Prostate cancer, then, is a mimic variant of the normal prostate gland tissue. Normal tissue cells reproduce themselves with remarkable fidelity. But, along the way, errors occur and are passed on, most of them unimportant. Usually, cells with such minor errors are removed by the body's immune system. Scientists now believe that virtually all tumors are monoclonal in origin, meaning that they are deviant "daughter" cells, descended from a "parent" cell, that contains DNA errors and have not been removed by normal processes. The damaged cells may have mutated many times along the way.

Cancer is deviant because it lacks the normal mechanisms that restrain cell growth in normal cells. Thus, tumor tissue is disordered, genetically unstable, and exhibits uncontrolled cell growth. Cancer cells do not have a normal cell's regulation mechanism. Ultimately, tumors impair the functioning of the original organ from which they descended.

The degree or amount of difference between the normal prostate tissue and the tumor tissue in any particular tumor cell is an indication of how virulent or "aggressive" your tumor is. This atypical cellular structure shows the pathologist how rapidly the tumor is growing.

Prostate cancer can vary from being almost benign to being quite aggressive. Unfortunately, medical science cannot tell us for sure which patient will do well with a minimal treatment and which of us could die without receiving aggressive intervention, such as surgery or radiation.

Obviously, prostate cancer presents your doctor or pathologist with a rather complex picture. There is more about this in the next three chapters, which discuss PSA, tumor grading, and staging.

Cancer of any kind is a complicated condition, and prostate cancer is no exception. There is no single ideal way to treat it. Since the condition itself is so variable and complicated, there are many treatment possibilities. This situation often puzzles the physician and can lead him astray in his original diagnosis. And since there are so many fields of treatment, there is competition among treatment practices. A particular physician prefers a given treatment because of his or her own training, experiences, and interpretation of the medical literature.

But, each specialist has chosen his field because of his experience and because he believes in his particular method. He thinks that he has done the thinking and evaluating for you, and you should reach the same conclusion he did. The truly open-minded physician will recommend that his patient investigate *all* approaches, because the physician alone cannot truly know what is "best" for a particular patient. He can advise, inform or suggest, but *you* have to decide.

The correct evaluation and treatment solution is seldom as clear-cut as is laid out in this guide. But, what follows should be useful as a *foundation* on which to form a treatment rationale for your own particular situation.

Remember This

Prostate cancer is not a communicable disease and the often used word "epidemic" is not appropriate. Prostate cancer is a condition of heredity, diet, environment, maleness, and aging. It is something we all face as we age. You will be overwhelmed with information regarding your condition and what to do about it, but there are only a dozen or so basic things you need to know about prostate cancer,

and this guide concentrates on those basics. Books cited in the bibliography can educate you further.

A crucial first step is to learn about your condition. The appendices in this guide contain many references to sources that will help educate you for the task ahead. Studies show that the most successful patients are those who take charge of the situation. These patients have better survival statistics, fewer side effects from treatment, and quicker, more complete recoveries. The goal of this book is to empower you with the basic information you must know as you confront a confusing and often frightening situation.

With early detection and intervention, it is an easy task to identify those men who are at high risk and treat them aggressively. The time will come when routine testing and a more aggressive attitude regarding early treatment will drastically reduce the death rate, and those 27,000 deaths per year will no longer mock us and threaten us. No man ought to die of prostate cancer.

Chapter 4

First Step: PSA

The very first information you need to know about *your* particular clinical condition is the type or grade of cancer you have, the tumor stage or physical extent of that tumor, and your Prostate Specific Antigen (PSA) value. You must request this information from your physicians. Learn what it means and master the implications of those numbers. Once you absorb these facts, you can start your own treatment tradeoff study. Every step of your journey will be governed by these numbers.

In this chapter and the two that follow I will begin to use more technical medical terminology to describe cancer conditions. I want to keep things simple and readable and not throw the reader off course with complex terminology or too much detail. This is difficult. Nevertheless, you will be rewarded if you take a little extra time with these chapters to familiarize yourself with the terminology. Much of what follows is dependent upon these concepts. Some of the terminology that you will encounter may be unfamiliar or downright confusing. The glossary at the end of this book provides a fuller description of the terms you will encounter in the text and hear from your physicians.

While the purpose of this guide is to show the treatment choices you have before you, *you do not have a completely free hand* in the choice of therapies available to you. The three principal numbers— cancer grade, stage, and PSA—combined with your age and level of health, will determine to a large extent which treatment pathways are open in your particular situation. After you determine the appropriate options open to you, you can decide on your personal preference for treatment.

There is some difficulty here as physicians (and the Treatment Option Charts) tell us that, since there are many ways to "skin a cat," no one can fully predict how a particular patient will fare with any particular treatment method.

Among several acceptable treatments, it comes down to the patient's choice 99 percent of the time. The Treatment Option Charts will assist you in making this crucial choice, one that is the most comfortable for you and will yield satisfactory results.

During the search for my own treatment choice, I talked with dozens of men who had already received treatment of some kind: surgery, radiation, seed implantation, cryosurgery. I was shocked that the majority of men I spoke to had no idea what is meant by Gleason grade or tumor stage. Most of them had a vague knowledge of their PSA numbers, but few had a grasp of what this number really meant. It is shocking to me that men can make life-altering decisions without knowing the critical factors that govern the decision-making process.

Let's start with the PSA diagnostic system. Most likely your cancer was indicated by this simple blood test, perhaps in conjunction with your physician's digital rectal exam (DRE). Many physicians and clinics are finally recognizing the value of this tool for prostate cancer diagnosis.

Chapter 5 will tell you about tumor grading and discuss the kinds of cancer that can develop. Chapter 6 will discuss the extent, or stage, of tumor development and what that implies regarding your treatment. You will see how the PSA level can correlate to both the type of tumor and the size of a developing tumor.

Prostate Specific Antigen is an organic glyco-protein that is made by the prostate and emitted into the blood stream. PSA is made only by prostate tissue and by no other tissue in the body. Normal prostates emit such tiny amounts of this chemical that it takes sophisticated laboratory testing equipment to detect it. It is measured in units of nanograms per milliliter of blood, that is to say in billionths of a gram in each few drops of blood.

In the past decade or so, it was discovered that the amount of this compound that is emitted into the blood stream is proportional to prostate activity. Malignant prostate cancer cells can produce more than ten times the amount of PSA per gram of tissue than is produced by normal tissue. Thus, an elevated PSA level is a warning that non-normal activity, such as would be produced by a beginning cancer, is taking place in the prostate. This does not mean that every man with an elevated PSA reading has prostate cancer. Elevations can occur because of benign prostatic hypertrophy, also called benign prostatic hyperplasia (BPH), a non-cancerous swelling that many men experience as they age. For those who have both BPH and cancer, the portion of PSA that was contributed by the cancer alone can confuse the issue further. Some 20 percent of normal prostates emit slightly elevated PSA, a fact that further complicates the picture.

In addition, inflammations of the prostate, called "prostatitis," can elevate PSA levels. There are a number of causes of prostatitis, and at one time or another most of us will have some degree of prostatitis, perhaps without even being aware of it.

If you have "normal" BPH as a result of aging, it is important to remember that there is some evidence that men with significant BPH have an increased risk of cancer. This possibility is still being investigated and debated, but it makes sense to approach the condition with caution and alertness.

More and more confidence is being built up regarding the accuracy of PSA analysis and its importance in discovering cancer early. Annual blood tests that present a consistently rising PSA number ought to merit further watching, more frequent blood testing, and perhaps biopsy examination of the prostate.

In addition to infection and BPH, PSA levels seem to be dependent upon age, and the size of the prostate. Physicians have developed new methods to track and interpret the results of PSA exams. Detection and interpretation of the results are improved by monitoring the annual *changes* of PSA levels (the velocity of change from year to year), assessing the PSA level in relation to the *size* of the prostate (the PSA "density"), adjusting to the patient's *age* (age-specific PSA), and the relationship of two types of PSA in the blood stream, the "free" PSA and the "bound" PSA, expressed as a *ratio*.

Scientists are now learning what levels of age-related PSA serve as a warning sign once they are exceeded. The following is a rough guide.

Age	**PSA Level**
40 – 50	2.5 ng/ml
50 – 60	3.5 ng/ml
60 – 70	4.5 ng/ml
70 – 80	6.5 ng/ml
80 +	? ?

Table 2
PSA versus Age

This table is only a convenience because the PSA values also relate to the size of a man's prostate. Large prostates produce more PSA than do smaller ones. So, your physician will consider your "prostate density" (defined as PSA per gram of prostate tissue), once he determines the volume of your gland with a sonogram image. He may adjust your PSA value accordingly. Normally he divides the raw PSA level by the prostate volume to obtain a ratio. Many believe a PSA *density* greater than 0.15 may indicate the presence of cancer.

You can see how this table relates to Table 1, Prostate Cancer and Aging, as shown in the Chapter 1.

There is serious debate in the oncology field about the

use of widespread PSA testing. You will probably hear about these arguments. Despite the conclusions of the Canadian study mentioned in Chapter 1, many physicians do not recommend widespread use of PSA testing, preferring instead to use it in a more limited way.

It is undeniable that PSA testing finds tumors earlier than in the past and that thousands of men might be saved by this testing. But, many argue that unnecessary trauma would result from indiscriminate use of this testing procedure. The argument is that many men, even if they *do* have cancer, need no treatment at all. And since the testing results are not 100 percent accurate, many men will suffer emotional trauma from false-positive and false-negative PSA results. Furthermore, the National Cancer Institute claims that sections of the country that rely heavily on PSA testing may have no greater success in reducing cancer deaths than areas that use PSA testing the least. Biopsy procedures subject men and insurance companies to financial costs that may not be necessary. Finally, early detection of prostate cancer will benefit a man only if the treatment is ultimately successful in prolonging the patient's life.

Many physicians believe that treatments for prostate cancer do not solve the problem. They believe that treatment itself might be worse for you than just leaving the cancer alone, that the quality of life you will experience after treatment is worse than it would be if you allowed the cancer to run its course.

Because of these and other arguments, even the National Cancer Institute, the American College of Physicians, and the American College of Preventive Medicine do not fully endorse wide-spread PSA screening . The American Cancer Society and the American Urological Association now recommend that high-risk men and men older than 50 be given this screening test and that they should be provided with information regarding risks and benefits of treatment if cancer is found.

I suppose that one could also make similar arguments against routine colonoscopy exams. I know several gastroenterologists who believe that with five-year colonoscopy screenings the incidence of fatal colon cancer would plummet. This cancer could be removed from the nation's statistical tabulation. I believe that the arguments against PSA screening support the financial aspects of our hospital and medical care infrastructure. I believe that screening for early detection of prostate cancer will result in the reduction of, if not the complete elimination of, death from prostate cancer.

Most doctors who oppose widespread screening limit their testing to high-risk patients. Patients who have a positive digital rectal exam, have families with a history of prostate cancer, or are African-American men over age 50, would be routinely tested. This is a kind of selective patient screening for PSA.

In late 1998 researchers at the Memorial Sloan-Kettering Cancer Center published new findings regarding a protein labeled p27. It is now believed that this protein plays a role in the development of many cancers, including prostate cancer. The researchers hope to be able to use this marker to predict whether the patient carries a slow-growing tumor or an aggressive or virulent type. Perhaps this development will help resolve the PSA controversy in the future and make screening more clear-cut.

If your PSA rises above the normal level for your age bracket, it is wise to obtain a further PSA analysis, but be sure it is done at a laboratory that has the *ultrasensitive* PSA methods. These newer techniques can obtain very accurate PSA levels. In the absence of BPH, a level of 10 ng/ml ought to be considered by everyone the point at which further testing is mandatory. Sonogram, MRI, CAT scan, or needle biopsy tests ought to be done. PSA numbers at this level, in the absence of BPH, are almost guaranteed to predict that you are developing a significant, clinically important tumor. Investigators have discovered that approximately 80 percent of men with elevated PSA levels have a clinically significant tumor. Indeed, there is clinical evidence that pre-treatment PSA levels greater than 20 ng/ml are associated with an increased risk of distant metastasis—or the spread of cancer to other parts of the body.

When a physician considers the *rate* that the PSA level rises from year to year as we age (the PSA velocity) he knows that PSA values rise more rapidly over time in men with prostate cancer than in men who are free from cancer. An increase greater than 0.75 ng/ml per year is regarded as an early warning predictor for cancer and may rule out the possibility that an increased PSA value is due solely to BPH or some other benign cause. Obviously it takes several years of testing in order to reach such a conclusion. Patients with elevated PSA levels that are stable and do not rise over time can be viewed with less concern by their physicians.

Finally, there are two types of Prostate Specific Antigen, the free PSA and the bound PSA. The free PSA is unbound to proteins and circulates in your blood stream unconnected to other proteins. Recent studies show that men with prostate cancer have a lower percentage of free PSA, and a higher percentage of bound PSA than men with prostatitis or BPH. This distinction will be useful to your physician, especially if he is unable to obtain a clear determination by his DRE. Most likely your PSA tests reported the total PSA value. If this number exceeds the age-related level shown in Table 2, you will want to order this ultrasensitive free and bound PSA analysis. By making an assessment of the *ratio* of free vs. bound PSA in your blood, your doctor can avoid unnecessary biopsies. If the ratio is below 14 percent, he will want to administer sonogram and needle biopsy procedures.

Before the introduction of PSA testing as a regular annual test, most prostate cancers were detected by digital rectal exams. When found by this method the tumors were usually advanced, and, therefore, more difficult to treat successfully. This fact is often overlooked in statistical studies of detection and treatment prior to 1990. With the widespread use of PSA testing, many more patients are being diagnosed far earlier than in the past, are receiving treatment earlier than in the past, and enjoy improved treatment outcomes.

PSA testing will continue to play a very important role in your life *after* you obtain treatment. Then it will serve as a monitoring device, the best indicator of possible residual tumor activity. The difficulty for any physician is that no matter what treatment you receive he cannot verify for sure that he has killed or removed every cancer cell in your body. The new ultrasensitive PSA assays turn positive when a patient has from 10,000 to 100,000 cancer cells at work. The fact is, depending upon your age and health, you may not have to remove all cancer cells from your body. If you live a normal life-span with no distress from cancer, you ought to consider that you have been cured, even though there are a few tumor cells left in your body. Most physicians consider your treatment a success if the "silent interval" for prostate cancer is longer than your remaining life span. By this reckoning, the definition of "cure" is altered from being cancer-free to being cancer distress-free.

Figure 3, from *The Prostate Forum*, Vol. 3, 1998, indicates the path that 30 doublings of an original cancer cell take to reach one billion cells, or a PSA value of about 3000. The graph shows the "silent interval" well. And it shows how long one may live with an active tumor, depending upon its aggressiveness, or doubling time.

Since the amount of PSA in your system is proportional to the size of your prostate and to the size and aggressiveness of a tumor, the doubling time of the PSA value will be significant to your physician. There is a tendency for Gleason grades to correlate to tumor doubling times. Low grade, well-differentiated tumors double in size slowly, while the higher grade, poorly-differentiated tumors have more rapid doublings. The PSA doubling time, therefore, will play a role in treatment choice, especially if the patient is considering a watchful waiting therapy.

After a radical prostatectomy your PSA levels should drop to zero. A level above 0.4 ng/ml may indicate residual cancer. And after radiation, if it doesn't drop to near zero, it ought to drop to insignificant levels. Levels above 0.5 ng/ml after radiation suggest recurrence of cancer. If measurable PSA numbers exist after such treatments it could mean that your cancer had escaped from the prostate prior to treatment and was missed by the therapy.

Thus, you can look at PSA testing first as a life saver for having discovered the presence of cancer early, and second as verifying that your physician has successfully removed cancer from your system. PSA testing will remain with you for the rest of your life. You and your physician will want to verify annually, or perhaps more frequently, that you are completely free of cancer.

Remember This

Prostate cancer, if found early, is entirely treatable. The key word is "early."

A recent randomized study conducted by Dr. F. Labrie in Quebec showed that men who were screened for early detection and who had aggressive treatment were more than 50 percent less likely to die of the condition. Early screening and detection is important in saving lives, and early detection is best done by PSA screening. And, of course, a new patient whose tumor is discovered early in its growth cycle has the most promising prognosis for his future.

I believe the arguments against screening for men above age 50 (and for higher risk men above 40), are unethical. Most educated or affluent men will get the screening

routinely in their annual physical exams. So, to deny testing to men who do not know about this subject is to engage in social and class discrimination. These are the men who are most likely to develop metastasized cancer without knowing it.

Chapter 5

Gleason Tumor Grading and Scoring

The type of cancer you have is determined by a biopsy (sample removal of tissue) and studies done under a microscope.

You need to know three things about the type or "grade" of cancer you have:

1. There are five common types of prostate cancer. Scientists *grade* them one through five. The most common type is type 3. Types 1 and 2 are quite slow growing, almost benign. If you are an 80-year-old man with either of these types, you can almost forget about treatment. Other health and aging factors will cause your death long before your cancer can grow to the point of danger.

But if you are type 4 or 5, then you must take action soon. These two types are considered very aggressive.

2. These five types are then "scored" with a scale called the Gleason *score*. Here, in addition to the basic grade type, 1 through 5, the second most prevalent cell grade in the biopsy sample is factored into the scoring system. My primary cell type was type 3, but the second most prevalent cell type was also type 3, so my final Gleason score was 6, a fairly common Gleason score. If my second most prevalent cancer grade had been a 4, my Gleason score would have been 7. Gleason scores range from 2 through 10. These are the numbers you will encounter in your reading, in discussions with your physicians and in the charts presented in this guide.

In your reading you will find the phrases "well-differentiated," "moderately-differentiated," and "poorly-differentiated." These phrases refer to the histological grade of your tumor cells, the degree of "togetherness" that the cancer cells present to the pathologist, and the associated Gleason type or grade numbers. Well-differentiated cells usually yield Gleason scores 2 to 4, which means that the tumor cells very closely resemble the normal prostate tissue. That is, the tumor glandular formation is very close to normal gland cells in appearance under the microscope. This is important because well-differentiated tumors have slow doubling times and respond nicely to treatment. These cancers have the lowest Gleason scores possible.

Moderately-differentiated cells yield Gleason scores 5 through 7, meaning the difference between normal prostate tissue and the tumor tissue is greater than in lower grade tissue. Most men fall into this tumor category. Correct grading is very important. It is sad, but true, that many pathologists don't know how to determine Gleason grades and scores accurately. It is important for you to have a second pathologist review your slides and the conclusions of the original pathologist.

An additional difficulty in grading comes from clinical evidence indicating that needle biopsies often underestimate the severity of the patient's cancer. That is, after a complete prostate is examined post-surgically, it is often found that a higher tumor grade existed than was estimated from the smaller needle samples previously available.

Poorly-differentiated cells are associated with Gleason scores 8 through 10, and involve the most virulent types or grades of tumor. If you have such a score, it means you cannot rely upon watchful waiting or delay your treatment for very long. Doubling time is far more rapid in this type of tumor.

You will also run across the term "ploidy" in your readings. This is a method of grading the DNA in your tumor cells. It reflects the derangement of cancer cells in your tumor. The chromosomes of cancer cells often are jumbled and in disarray.

There are three ploidy terms that pathologists use in this measurement, and you may see them mentioned in your biopsy reports. Diploid cancer cells have the normal number of chromosomes and are usually less difficult to treat, as they are most likely slow growing and will not spread easily. Diploid tumors are the most common ploidy pattern found in all prostate cancers, regardless of stage. Aneuploid cells behave more aggressively and do not respond as easily to treatment, because of the disruption of the chromosomes. Thus, a tumor with a high percentage of aneuploid cells presents some treatment difficulties that your doctor would not have to consider if the percentage were low or absent. Higher percentages of aneuploid cells mean that you should not choose a watch and wait treatment. Tetraploid cells are between diploid and aneuploid types. The pathologist who examines your biopsy material will state a percentage of the various types of ploidy. Usually a tumor contains more than one type of ploidy cells .

3. The type of cancer you have will most likely stay the same and will *not* evolve into one of the more aggressive types. So, on learning that you are a grade 3, do not make the common emotional conclusion of saying, "Gad, I'm already a 3 and will soon be a 4 or 5!" Prostate cancer of a Gleason grade 3 will probably remain at this grade even if it spreads to your bones or organs.

But there is discussion on this latter point. There is some, as yet inconclusive, evidence that some cancers can "de-differentiate" and become more aggressive over time. Right now there is no real proof of a definite progression of well-differentiated (low Gleason grade) cancer into a higher grade tumor. Such a thesis is difficult to prove at this time. However, some physicians believe that this can occur.

Remember This

The type or grade of cancer you have is a key diagnostic factor in determining your ultimate treatment and the urgency for your treatment. This factor is so important that

it is wise to have several treatment centers review your biopsy slides so that the scoring is verified.

Chapter 6

Staging

Most men do not have prostate cancer per se. They have prostate cancers, meaning there are usually a number of centers from which larger tumors grow.

Tumor staging refers to the size and location of the tumor and whether or not it has escaped the prostate. How big is it? Can it be felt by the digital rectal examination? If not, it is "staged" as a T1 tumor. If it can be felt by the DRE, you are staged a T2 or higher. More than 25 percent of initial diagnoses are in the T2 stage. How much of the prostate is affected by the tumor? Clinical evidence suggests that about 85 percent of men with a tumor have multiple tumor sites within the prostate.

Has tumor material spread to locations outside but near the prostate? If so, you are staged as a T3. About 30 percent of initial diagnoses are stage T3. A T3 stage situation means that radiation may be involved, as surgical removal of the entire prostate is unlikely to remove all tumor material from your body.

A T4 stage, which is rare, means that the cancer is outside the prostate and has metastasized or spread to other areas of the body. In such a case the treatment procedures will be completely different than would be the case for patients with a lesser stage. While surgery or radiation may be useful, the main treatment focus here will involve hormonal control, orchiectomy, or chemotherapy.

Staging is a partially subjective measure and has its flaws, but is very important, even with its inaccuracies. You will see many articles and tables that use this staging system. In fact, staging is as important as tumor grade and PSA level in assessing your true condition. Clinically, the most important break point is between stages T1/T2 and stages T3/T4.

Accurate staging is very important in determining the proper treatment, even though more and more men are being diagnosed "by accident" via needle biopsy, and are technically in the non-alarming T1 category.

Several other systems indicate staging. You will find these in your readings; many doctors still refer to them. In order to be clear about these, the following comparison table shows how the numbers work and what they mean to you. In this book I will use the newer TNM International Staging System (which is replacing the old Whitmore-Jewett A,B,C,D Staging System). T stands for tumor (with the various sub-numbers representing size and extent of the tumor), N stands for lymph nodes (and tells us if the cancer has spread to them, (0 or 1, or +), and M indicates that it is metastatic, having spread to distant locations of the body, (0 or 1, or +).

TNM System	Whitmore - Jewett System	Description
T0		No tumor evidence
Stage 1	**Stage A**	Clinical suspicion of tumor development
T1a	A1	Microscopic tumor site(s) usually well-differentiated
T1b	A2	Multiple foci and less well-differentiated
T1c	B0	Tumor confirmed by needle biopsy. Elevated PSA
Stage 2	**Stage B**	Tumor present and limited to prostate
T2a	B1	Small tumor, one lobe of prostate. DRE now positive
T2b	B2	Tumor size is greater than 1.5 cc
T2c	B3	Tumor on both lobes of prostate
Stage 3	**Stage C**	Tumor spreads outside of prostate
T3a	C1	One sided extracapsular spread
T3b	C2	Bilateral spread of tumor materials
T3c		Tumor has spread into seminal vesicles
Stage 4	**Stage D**	Cancer has spread to lymph nodes or beyond
T4a	D1	Cancer has spread to bladder neck, sphincter, or rectum
T4b		Cancer has spread to elevator muscles or pelvic wall
	D2	Distant metastases
Lymph node metastases		
N0		No lymph node involvement
N1	D1	Lymph nodes less than 2 cm in diameter
N2		One node greater than 2 cm but less than 5 cm
N3		Lymph node(s) greater than 5 cm
Distant Metastases		
M0		No distant metastases
M1a	D2	Lymph nodes other than adjacent nodes
M1b		Skeletal involvement
M1c		Other sites
	D3	Cancer is resistant to hormonal therapy

Table 3
Prostate Cancer Staging Systems

There are some problems with these staging systems because they are somewhat subjective. Prior to surgery it is difficult to tell with certainty whether a cancer is truly confined to the prostate. There is always a chance of "extracapsular penetration," or "extension," by the tumor. These terms indicate that the cancer is escaping beyond the prostate walls, and that it may be about to spread to other areas of your body. Staging numbers always have this uncertainty to them.

Confident staging and treatment recommendations will be rare because of the differences of opinion among physicians. One clinician may differ from another as a result of his individual experience. Indeed, many physicians do not even recognize the T2c or T3c category shown in the table. Others find these categories useful.

The difficulty in determining the correct stage of your tumor and whether it is an organ-confined or a metastasized condition will cause you some concern. Confident and assured resolution of this problem should not be expected, as there is no clear-cut line between staging categories. Rather, there is a continuous gradation of tumor growth progress.

Clinical staging is the estimate arrived at after all non-invasive methods of examination have been considered. The stage value that your physicians apply to you is an *estimate* of how much cancer is in your body and where it is located.

The true *pathologic* condition can be determined only after removal of the prostate. When prostate surgery is performed, the surgeon will remove the gland intact and he will also take samples of the nearby lymph nodes and seminal vesicles. These tissues will be sent to the laboratory for examination by pathologists. They will make the biopsy examination of the margins of the prostate, the seminal vesicles, the lymph nodes, etc. Without this physical evidence, staging estimates will vary among physicians.

Statistical studies of surgeries show that more often than

not the original clinical stage value was incorrect, that it was originally "under-staged" by the physician. This means that your physician may have concluded from his DRE, imaging, and biopsy tests that your tumor was smaller than it really was, or had not penetrated the wall of your prostate when it really had. That is one reason that surgical removal of the entire prostate, when the tumor was originally judged to be "organ confined," has a high incidence of recurrence of cancer.

Laboratory pathology examinations show that approximately 40 percent to 50 percent of "organ-confined" prostates have tumors that were *not* confined to the prostate after all. Obviously, it is immensely important to have your condition accurately staged, because if you are understaged or undergraded, you may wind up not being treated correctly and completely.

The staging number is often modified to include a prefix of "c" or "p", indicating that the stage was determined "clinically" prior to surgery, or "pathologically" from studies made of the prostate after it is removed.

Thus, a patient designated as a cT2a is estimated to have a tumor on one side of his gland, the tumor being detectable with the DRE. But if the post-operative examination by the pathologist shows that the tumor has actually penetrated the prostate wall, or had invaded nearby tissue such as the seminal vesicles or the lymph nodes, he will re-stage the condition as a pT3a. You may discover such stage values in your reading.

Finally, it is important to your physician to know where within your prostate a tumor is located. Is it near the bladder or at the apex, or bottom, of the prostate? Such considerations may help decide whether surgery or radiation is the appropriate treatment option. Is the tumor in the central region of the prostate and unlikely to escape the prostate if you delay treatment? Is it in the transition zone of the prostate, or is it in the peripheral zone, where it is close to the prostate wall and offers a potential for escape? Your physician will be on the alert for such a possibility.

Figure 4 (see color section) is a tabulation of all the factors mentioned so far, factors that are important to you once you have been diagnosed with prostate cancer. It also illustrates the level of the risk associated with each factor, and the sum of these risk considerations may determine treatment urgency for you. A review of the definitions of the TNM staging system in Table 3 will help you fully understand this figure. You may wish to locate your condition in the various urgency categories. These factors will influence the treatment options available to you.

These options, and a number of factors associated with them, will influence your particular tradeoff rationale. This discussion is covered in the next chapter.

Remember This

Accurate staging assessment for each unique patient is perhaps the major factor in determining proper treatment.

Despite ambiguities in determining clinical stage values for a tumor, it is critically important to make the most accurate assessment as is possible. A patient would be wise to have several physicians make independent assessments of his staging. Sonogram procedures will help here so that visual images can be examined. An array of sonogram-guided needle biopsies could also help delineate the amount of tumor material inside the prostate.

In an as yet unpublished study (as of March 1999), Dr. Mack Roach at the UCSF Medical Center, reviewed case histories of some 1500 prostate cancer patients across the nation. His findings indicate that only three significant factors determine whether or not a patient will die of the condition: Gleason score, advanced stage, and lymph node

involvement.

In order for you to determine an appropriate treatment for your specific situation, you need to know your Gleason grade and score, the staging of your tumor, your PSA value, and whether or not the cancer is confined to the prostate gland. Without this knowledge you will have difficulty deciding what to do.

Chapter 7

The Tradeoff

Enlightened physicians will advise you to see a number of other physicians, especially those proficient in other treatment methodologies. It is wise to follow such a course, getting all the facts you can on the various procedures that are open to you.

And, if you are like me, you may experience a sense of relief and confidence after visits to various physicians. For instance, after interviewing a seed implantation radiologist, you may return home confident that this is the superior approach. Most likely you will hold this view until you talk with a cryosurgeon or a proton beam radiologist.

You will read books, and as fine as many of them are, your confusion may only be increased. In my own experience, I often reached the point of frustration and despair.

In order to reduce the emotional highs and lows during my search, I devised a number of treatment option decision tradeoff diagrams. I approached this task from three directions:

1. Which treatments were eligible or ineligible for consideration because of my particular tumor score, stage, PSA, age, and health statistics? To unravel this issue, I drew up my charts. After I did this, I was able to focus on the appropriate treatment possibilities open to me.

2. Which treatment offered the best mortality and morbidity statistics? The word "mortality" pertains to death statistics and what to expect long term. "Morbidity" defines health conditions that you do not now have, but that may result as a side effect, say, of radiation or surgery.

You should focus on the survival statistics not only for the long term, but for the short term as well. If surgery appeals to you, do you have any health conditions that could put you at risk of death with this approach? (There is a risk of death in any surgery.)

Does the issue of future incontinence bother you more than the issue of future impotence? I know a man who would have opted for no treatment so as to keep his sexuality intact, despite the prognosis of a very limited life-span if he remained untreated. For me this is incomprehensible. I concentrated on killing cancer cells as effectively as possible, keeping incontinence second to this and impotence third in my decision rationale. Impotence can be treated, and I reasoned that I would not be particularly sexually attractive to my wife if I were wearing diapers. The end of the world for me is death. But each man has to make his own decision. All therapies have these factors to consider, and each treatment results in different statistics for the four main concerns you ought to have right now:

Basic survival
Incontinence
Impotence
Secondary side effects, as defined by the Therapy Oncology Group (RTOG) listing of secondary side effects

Each man must decide his own order of importance for these issues.

The Radiation Therapy Oncology Group has designed a rating system to indicate the secondary morbidity conditions associated with various treatment procedures. You will find references to these "grades" in the literature you study. They are shown in Table 4.

You should discuss these conditions with each of your physicians. Make sure you understand this grading system and learn about the various minor conditions that are associated with the grading in the morbidity table. Compare these factors among the various treatment possibilities you have under consideration.

3. Lastly, I wanted to know which primary treatment compromised or closed any future treatment option in the

event of a failure with my primary treatment choice.

For instance, if you choose general X-ray radiation, will this result in closing the option for future X-ray treatments? Will it prevent surgery as a future treatment option? Which treatment option is closed to you (or may impair your future health or the effectiveness of a future treatment, if required) if you choose radioactive seed implantation?

If you are like me, you will wake up at night and experience a surge of anxiety or fear. Many times during your research, you will run into conflicting or disturbing information. You will be beset with doubts at times.

Grade	Symptoms
1	Minor symptoms requiring no corrective treatment.
2	Symptoms responding to simple outpatient management. Life style not affected.
3	Distressing symptoms altering patient's life style. Hospitalization for diagnosis or minor surgical intervention (such as urethal dilation) may be required.
4	Major surgical intervention (such as laparoscopy, colostomy, cystectomy) or prolonged hospitalization.
5	Fatal Complications.

Table 4
RTOG Morbidity Grading System

Consult your tradeoff Treatment Option Charts for reassurance that *you* are obtaining the relevant information and that you are processing it intelligently. This will help you gain control of your emotions. This knowledge will prevent cancer from controlling your emotions and your life.

The majority of men are diagnosed with prostate cancer that is slow growing. Each treatment option has various side effects, any of which may decrease your quality of life. In the long run, each of us must make his own treatment tradeoff decision. In searching for your most satisfying option, you may be tapping your deepest resources.

The Treatment Option Decision Charts and the treatment chapters that follow may help illuminate this search for you. Keep in mind that you have some other considerations to weigh. These are treatment location and lodgings if away from home. Hospitalization time, time away from work, and physical changes to your life during convalescence are also of concern. Each treatment chapter provides a brief idea of what to expect. While you should not allow these considerations to unduly influence your treatment determination, the guide lets you know at least a bit about what to expect.

Remember This

Your specific medical conditions play an important role in finding the appropriate treatment option for you. Once those treatment options are determined, your choice will depend upon the mortality and morbidity numbers that will affect your quality of life after treatment.

These statistics relate to your initial survival of the treatment, future incontinence, impotence, and a number of secondary side effects caused by the treatment.

Finally, before you decide upon your primary treatment option, you will want to consider the subject of future treatment options open to you in the event of a recurrence of your cancer.

Chapter 8

Statistics

If you are like I am, you avoided the subject of statistics when you were in school. As a science student, I was forced to study the subject more than I wished, finding it tedious and boring. It is boring no longer, because the statistics for my cancer, my treatment choice, and my present quality of life touch me daily. You, too, will face these basic statistics, and they will impact your life from now on.

Beware! The statistics you encounter regarding treatment and future quality of life may or may not be true.

You need to know your important statistics, and what they mean. They affect survival and the quality of life you will experience after treatment of any kind. Approximately 50 percent of prostate cancer patients indicate that preservation of their quality of life is the most important consideration to them. The critical categories to consider are:

Mortality: Whether or not you will survive the treatment process.

Survival Period: The length of time you will probably live after treatment. This is based upon the clinical histories of thousands of patients. The literature presents statistics on "disease specific survival rates," and "overall survival rates." You will see charts showing these outcomes, and those charts may cause you some alarm. The first one relates to patient death *because* of prostate cancer, and the second relates to patient death after treatment, but from *all* possible causes. You must be able to distinguish between these concepts.

Morbidity: Statistics relating to the quality of life conditions that are caused by the treatment process. The two most important issues are incontinence, and impotence, although there is a host of lesser conditions that can be more than mere annoyances. (See Table 4).

Recurrence Rate: The chances that your primary treatment will be unsuccessful and that your cancer will recur.

Typically, you will see data for five-year and ten-year periods.

Figure 9 gives you a rough comparison for these important categories of clinically reported statistics and how they may affect future treatment options open to you in case the primary treatment fails.

Although there are many fine surgeons and radiologists operating outside the country's major clinics, you should realize that the mortality, survival, and morbidity statistics that you read about and discuss with your physicians were gathered from the big clinics. A moment's reflection will suggest that those numbers are too optimistic, perhaps much too optimistic.

In an as yet unpublished study conducted by Dr. Mack Roach at UCSF Medical Center, he showed that even agreement among pathologists examining microscope slides of tumor material is poor. That is, the pathologists outside of major clinical institutions are unable to agree with something as basic as the scoring determined by pathologists at major centers. He stresses that a critical aspect of patient success is to guarantee that the scoring is accurate.

The numbers reported in books and in this guide are taken from data reported by the country's *first-rate clinics,* and do not reflect the overall average that would include data from all hospitals and treatment centers in the nation. It would be impossible for anyone to compile the true statistics. But, as a starting point, US-TOO International, Inc. has a report titled *Perspectives on Prostate Cancer Treatments, A Study of Patients and Urologists*, conducted by pollster Louis Harris in 1995. This report presents highlights of the survey on the impact of prostate cancer on patient's lives, and compares the responses to questions given by patients and the perceptions of their doctors. There are many insights here, and you will be educated by this report, even though it is several years old. When you consider your options, quality of life and recurrence rates, do so with the understanding that you are looking at the most optimistic numbers available.

You may find a surgeon, for instance, who can improve on those numbers. The law of averages, however, suggests that you will find a surgeon whose record is not as good as those shown in the literature.

To help solve this question, consider taking your own quality of life survey of prostate cancer survivors. Forget the published statistics. What would cancer survivors *themselves* tell you about the choices they made in their treatment? What would they say about their post-treatment quality of life? What would they say about the correctness of their original treatment decision? Are they satisfied or unhappy with the path they followed? While this hypothetical poll is impossible to conduct nationwide, you can obtain such insights at your local level by joining a nearby prostate cancer support group.

The place to begin this study is Appendix B, which lists a number of support group organizations and directories. Do this today!

If your physician places you on combined hormonal therapy, you will have time to weigh the evidence given by the others in your local support group. You will learn far more from even this limited sampling than you will by studying the statistics presented in the literature, and even perhaps, by listening to your own physician.

Many things are said, but unproven, with respect to quality of life issues post-surgery, post-radiation, and post-seed implantation therapy. My discussions on treatment with a dozen or more fellow patients showed me that the average patient was confused, ignorant, and frightened. A man may have gone to a local oncologist believing he has found a "good doctor," whatever that might mean. Conducting your own local poll will make you sensitive to the *real issue* before you: the quality of life you will have *after* your treatment for prostate cancer.

Remember This

The morbidity and other statistics published in journals and books are skewed. Taking into consideration all surgical operations and radiation treatments across the nation, the published numbers are far more optimistic than the average results.

The side effects that you have after surgery will most likely remain with you for the rest of your life. The side effects you have after radiation will most likely *worsen* as the years go by. Ultimately, you could face complete impotence as a result of radiation treatment.

Do not make any decision based upon the published numbers.

Do not hurry in making your final treatment decision.

Join your local prostate cancer support group to learn from the experiences of those in your immediate vicinity. You will get a valuable education by taking your own private poll. Learn as much as possible from men who have already gone through treatment and what their personal disappointments may be. This experience may help you a great deal in your own treatment decision.

Prostate cancer patients who are members of their local support group seem to do better than those who "go it alone." Being a member of your local support group will improve your outcome.

Chapter 9

Prostate Cancer Treatment Option Charts

Some books and articles on prostate cancer will clarify the subject for you; others will confuse you. Similarly, some doctors and clinicians will be decisive, while some will be evasive. Some will emphasize a particular aspect of your condition, while others may minimize that same point.

Some physicians will just plain mis-diagnose your clinical condition.

That is why I wrote at the beginning of this guide that you must learn the issues and deal with confusion and misunderstanding. The doctors themselves must deal with confusion, as there is still much to learn about prostate cancer and the most effective treatments for it. I had no idea there were so many treatment possibilities. Each treatment method competes in the marketplace against the others, competes for your pocketbook, competes for your mind and competes for your emotions. There is intense interest, as well as uncertainty, in both the scientific and lay communities, regarding the proper diagnosis and preferred treatment for prostate cancer.

This confusion is part of the environment you are now in. I have used my background in science and engineering to work out and visually display, in a systematic manner, the basic elements of concern. I hope that this approach will save you time, money, and emotional distress and that you will be able to see clearly the choices that lie before you.

I discovered that most publications on prostate cancer have so much information in them that the reader cannot absorb it. I believe that these books actually fail the reader because he will put the unreadable book aside and miss learning the few basics that he must know in order to arrive at an appropriate and confident treatment decision. In so doing, he fails to develop a positive sense that *he* is in control, and this is detrimental to his ultimate success. Most of the books and articles I studied are not recommended in this guide. I *do* recommend the books listed in the bibliography.

How *does* one sort out all the information, misinformation, conflicting opinions and confusion and arrive at a reasonable course of action? I began with rough charts and graphs. I sorted out the kind of tumor I was suspected of having, my clinical stage, what my PSA level meant, and factored in my age and general health. Then I was able to construct the Treatment Option Charts. Finally, I drew more charts to outline the course of future action in case the treatment I decided on turned out not to eliminate all the cancer.

The combination of these graphs, charts, and tables led me to a treatment path that had the greatest likelihood of bringing me a successful cure. At the same time, they showed me which options were still open if, for some reason, the primary treatment failed.

Before I was able to construct my Treatment Option Charts, I had to sort through a mass of conflicting information in an attempt to bring order out of chaos. I started by reading and by asking many questions of my physicians. Lists and lists of questions. I often thought that after I left my appointments my doctors were in need of a double scotch and soda. But only by investigation was I able to construct the charts and graphs and find my own way out of the information maze.

By doing this tedious exercise, I learned three important lessons:

1. I discovered what was important for my particular case and what to concentrate on in my reading.

2. I knew what questions to ask my physicians. I could now engage them as partners as we plotted our course of action. The Treatment Option Charts in this book may help guide you and your physician to the appropriate therapy for *your* particular situation. My goal is to let you find your

unique situation, so you can free your mind of the mass of data that confronts you.

3. By constructing the charts, I discovered that my anxieties almost disappeared. *I* was in control. Ultimately, I *knew* that I would be successfully cured. I felt that my treatment choice was well-founded and that, in the event of possible primary treatment failure, I knew what the next step would be for me. I learned what future therapy would be denied me if I chose one primary therapy over another. This knowledge assisted me in choosing the primary method in the first place.

I appeared for my treatment confident, relaxed, and self-possessed.

I hope that you do, too. I think it will help and calm you to spend some time with these charts and the explanations of them.

The following charts are not meant to be a cookbook answer for you. Nothing is absolute in this game, but they are a starting point for you. They are meant to be used as guides. If your urologist recommends something that seems inappropriate from your understanding of a potential treatment path, then you need to discuss his recommendation thoroughly with him, perhaps using the charts to broaden your discussions with him. These guides should give you confidence that you will find your way out of your dilemma and reach a successful conclusion.

Figure 5 introduces you to the basic treatment option decision approach. It shows how to use the Treatment Option Charts for the five types of prostate cancer. The varibles incorporated in these charts are:

Gleason Score (Remember that this score is the sum of the two prevalent tumor types or grades.)
Stage (The size or spread of the tumor.)
Age
Health

Note that the PSA level is left off these charts. It was one variable too many for me to display in a clear manner. This factor is usually associated with the staging decision anyway, and helps confirm the stage value that is assigned to the patient. Usually a low PSA value indicates a small tumor, while an elevated PSA value would verify a higher stage number.

The charts use a color scheme for treatment pathways. Green is used if you are in excellent health for your age, blue for average health, and red for poor health.

In the charts to come, you will encounter white circles, white squares, and white diamonds. The meaning of these symbols is as follows:

White circles identify a PRIMARY treatment option, defined as treatment expected to rid you of cancer.

White squares indicate treatments that are applied as CO-PARTNER or *adjuvant* therapy to the primary treatment, but do not rid you of cancer by themselves. Most of these therapies use hormone treatments as an adjunct to a primary treatment option, such as surgery or radiation. In coming years, combined hormonal therapies may be established as routine adjuvant/co-partners for all primary treatments.

White diamonds indicate the use of a primary treatment as a SECONDARY assist, which is defined as a treatment that will not eradicate cancer by itself, but may contribute to the effectiveness of the primary treatment. This treatment might have been considered as a primary treatment option in another case, but is used here only to shrink and control the main tumor. For instance, radiation to attack the main tumor is a possibility even in a T4 patient whose primary treatment is an orchiectomy, hormonal therapy, chemotherapy, or clinical trial, each of which is designed to focus on the metastasized targets elsewhere within the body.

The charts that follow have seven categories as target

therapies, and the numbering in the text and on the charts refers to these treatments:

Treatment Option No.	Treatment Option
1	Watchful waiting.
2	Watchful waiting combined with hormone therapies.
3	Surgery.
4	External beam radiation (EBRT).
5	Brachytherapy (Seed implantation).
6	Cryosurgery.
7	Chemotherapy, orchiectomy, alternate therapies, or clinical trials.

Table 5
Treatment Options

I realize that this is getting a bit complicated, but I have tried to construct the Treatment Option Charts as simply as possible, while staying true to the medical situation.

Let's go back a step and review the instructional chart on Figure 5, page 54. It is the instructional chart to Figures 6, 7, and 8, and tells you how to start your treatment discovery. Remember, to begin your assessment on Figures 6, 7 & 8, find your Gleason tumor score in the appropriate Treatment Options Chart, or in the left-hand column. Find your stage value in the next column, and then, working with your age group and health category, move to the right along the correct color bar until you find a white circle, square, or diamond. No doubt you will have several white indicators located in your particular color bar. These point to the primary treatment categories appropriate for you, (as well as to the adjuvant/co-partner therapies, and the secondary treatments), numbered at the top of the appropriate chart.

Now turn to Figures 6, 7, and 8. These Treatment Option Charts are the detailed guidelines for the five tumor grades: One and two (Gleason score of 2 to 4), three (Gleason score of five, six, and seven), and four and five (Gleason score of eight to ten). You will choose *one* of these charts, depending upon your Gleason score. *Ignore the other charts.* Each of these charts is subdivided into the stage of your tumor, T1, T2, T3, or T4. Your age and health statistics (in color) further delineate your options.

To find a treatment option that is appropriate for your particular Gleason score condition, simply identify your stage value, age, and health on one of the three charts. Then follow the colored bands to the white circle which indicates a primary therapy that is a possibility for you. In many cases, there are several treatments that could be appropriate. The final choice of treatment can then be decided upon in discussions with your physicians and by reviewing the information in Figure 9.

If you run into a white square, you have identified a primary treatment co-partner, or adjuvant therapy option, that your physician may wish to employ to assist the effectiveness of the primary treatment. If you run into a white diamond, this indicates a secondary treatment option which cannot be expected to cure you by itself, but may improve the ability of the primary treatment in its work.

The clustering of possible treatment options shifts from the upper left area of the charts to the lower right portion. You can see that if you are younger than sixty, in excellent health, and have a low grade tumor, you might go right to surgery, external beam radiation, or brachytherapy. Any of these treatments will give you an excellent chance of a full recovery.

However, if you are in poor health, over age 70, and have a stage T3 or T4 tumor with a Gleason score of 10, you can not rely upon any of the younger man's options. You are headed directly to chemotherapy, alternative therapies, clinical trials, or an orchiectomy, perhaps combining radiation or hormone treatments to retard, but not cure, your condition, as indicated by the white squares and diamonds.

I have mentioned that the proper treatment decision is not clear-cut, and this is especially true when you incorporate your age and health if your tumor stage is T3 or T4. You are outside the simpler T1/T2 bracket. Most likely you will use several treatment options in some combination. For instance, on Figure 8 you can see that the white circles for your primary treatment most likely cannot be expected to cure you of cancer completely. In most cases your physician will combine other options, probably treatment number 2, watchful waiting with hormones. But, in this case, the white square identifies the use of hormones no longer as a primary treatment but as an adjuvant/co-partner therapy to your primary white circle treatment number 7. A white diamond for a T3/T4 patient indicates the use of radiation to shrink the primary tumor so that the primary chemical treatment will be more effective. The medical profession is finding that the high risk patient who first undergoes radiation or surgical debulking of the prostate stands a better chance that his condition can be controlled than if he underwent only an orchiectomy, for instance.

For a low Gleason score patient with a T1/T2 stage category, the decision path is relatively easy, as shown in Figure 6. He will not require secondary assisting therapies. Such a patient, perhaps, may use hormones as a adjuvant/co-partner to his primary surgery or radiation treatments. Most patients whose cancer is discovered early will reside in this area, or in that of Figure 7.

Again, I stress that the Treatment Option Charts may be different from what your urologist tells you. Many urologists and physicians will argue the fine points, including the use of a radical prostatectomy for a T4 patient! Use these charts and tables to debate the fine points with your physicians.

Now, just as you are getting your fill of these charts I have one more for you! The final chart I call the "Future Treatment Options Chart." It is an inescapable fact that primary treatment is an inexact science, so we must accept the possibility that some tumors return. Thus, you must study which treatment options may be closed to you in the future if you choose one primary treatment over another. What options for future treatment do you eliminate by choosing a particular primary treatment? These considerations are outlined in Figure 9. When deciding between primary treatments with very similar survival statistics, the likely side effects and the future treatment options could be the determining factors for your primary choice. Use Figure 9 to find out what options are open, closed, or compromised in some way. Look at the clinical statistics concerning incontinence, impotence, and recurrence rates for each eligible primary treatment you consider.

In the case of primary treatment numbers 1 and 2, all future options remain open to you. In the case of treatment number 7, the more invasive treatments are just not appropriate to handle the stage that mandated this treatment option in the first place. With the exception of localized radiation treatments as an assist, they will not be effective in curing your cancer.

For primary treatments 3 through 6, the chart shows several possible side effects (such as incontinence and impotence) related to each treatment, in addition to which future treatment options are closed to you in case the cancer returns. Remember that these statistics are reported by large clinical centers and so tend to be more optimistic than a national average would be. Some options are still open, but they are compromised in some way, meaning that they come with significant difficulties that you need to inquire about before you choose your primary treatment. A choice

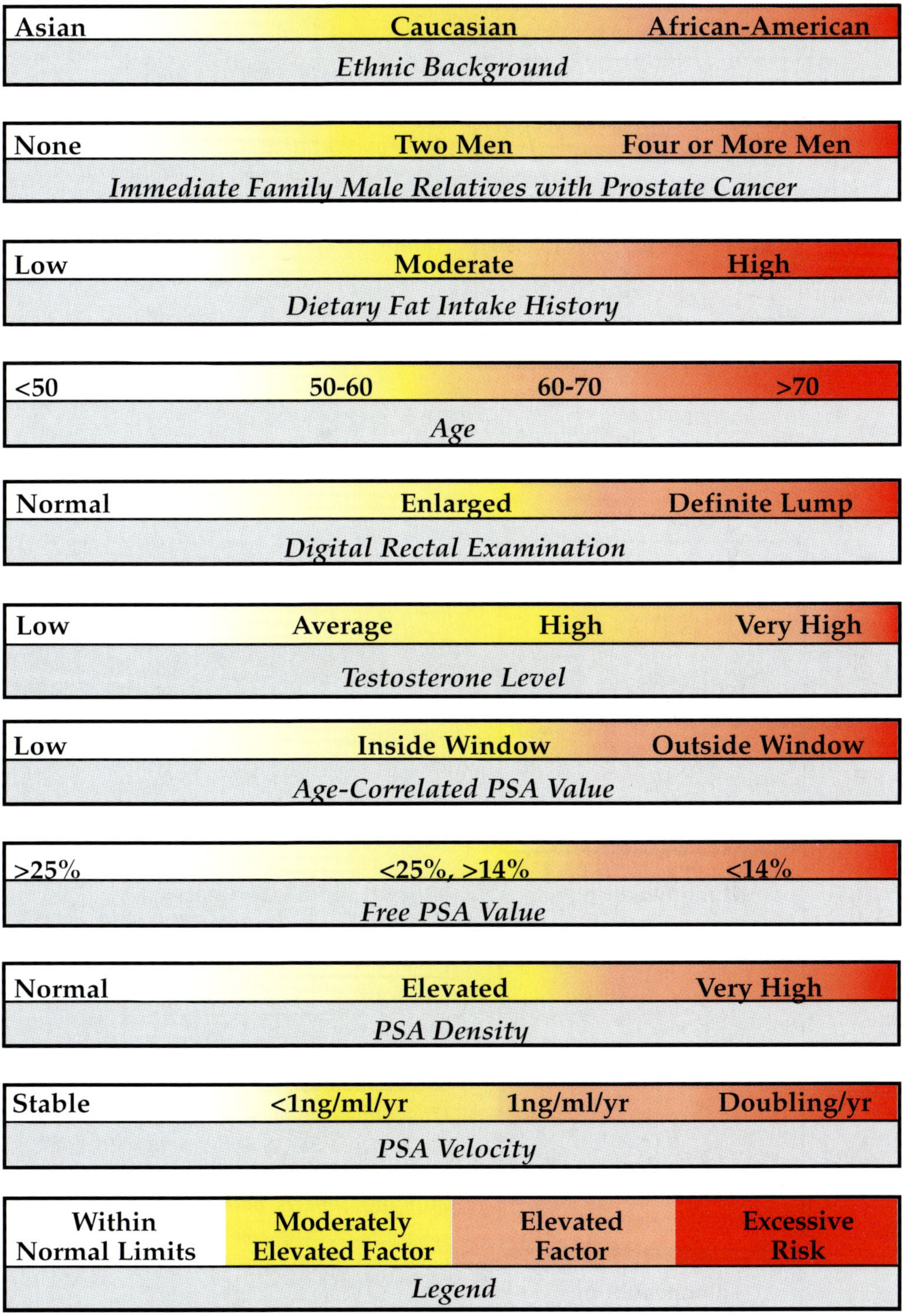

Figure 1

Pre-Diagnostic Factors for Elevated Risk

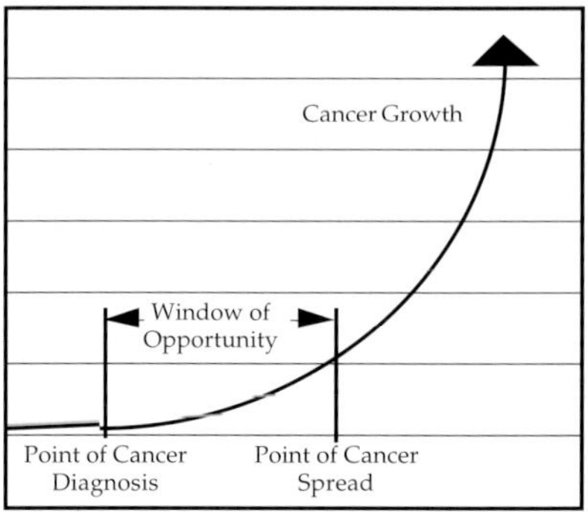

The time from diagnosis until the cancer has started to spread is called the window of opportunity. During this time curative treatment should be successful. The actual time within the window depends upon the aggressiveness of the particular tumor.

Figure 2
Window of Opportunity

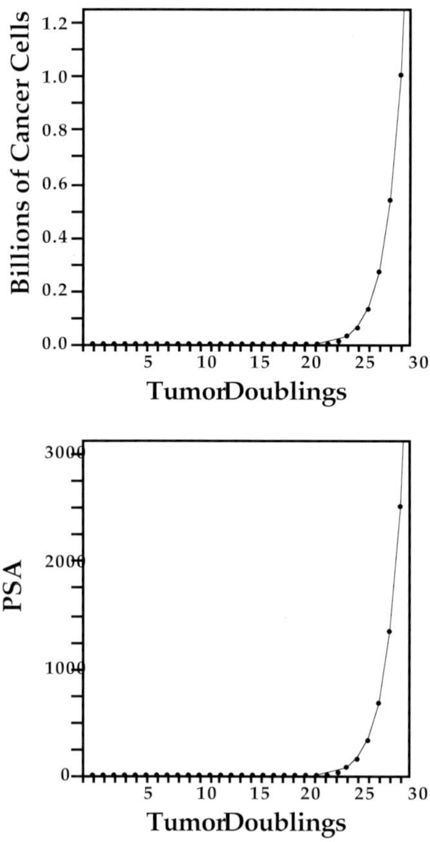

The top graph on the left starts with one cancer cell and follows it through 30 doublings. The bottom figure shows the approximate PSA values with each tumor doubling shown in the top curve.

Doubling Time	Time to Reach PSA of 1000
2 Weeks	5.5 Months
3 Months	2.75 Years
1 Year	11 Years
5 Years	55 Years

This table shows how long it takes to go from a PSA of 0.5 to close to 1000. The importance of a slow or rapid doubling time is obvious.

Figure 3
Tumor Doubling Times

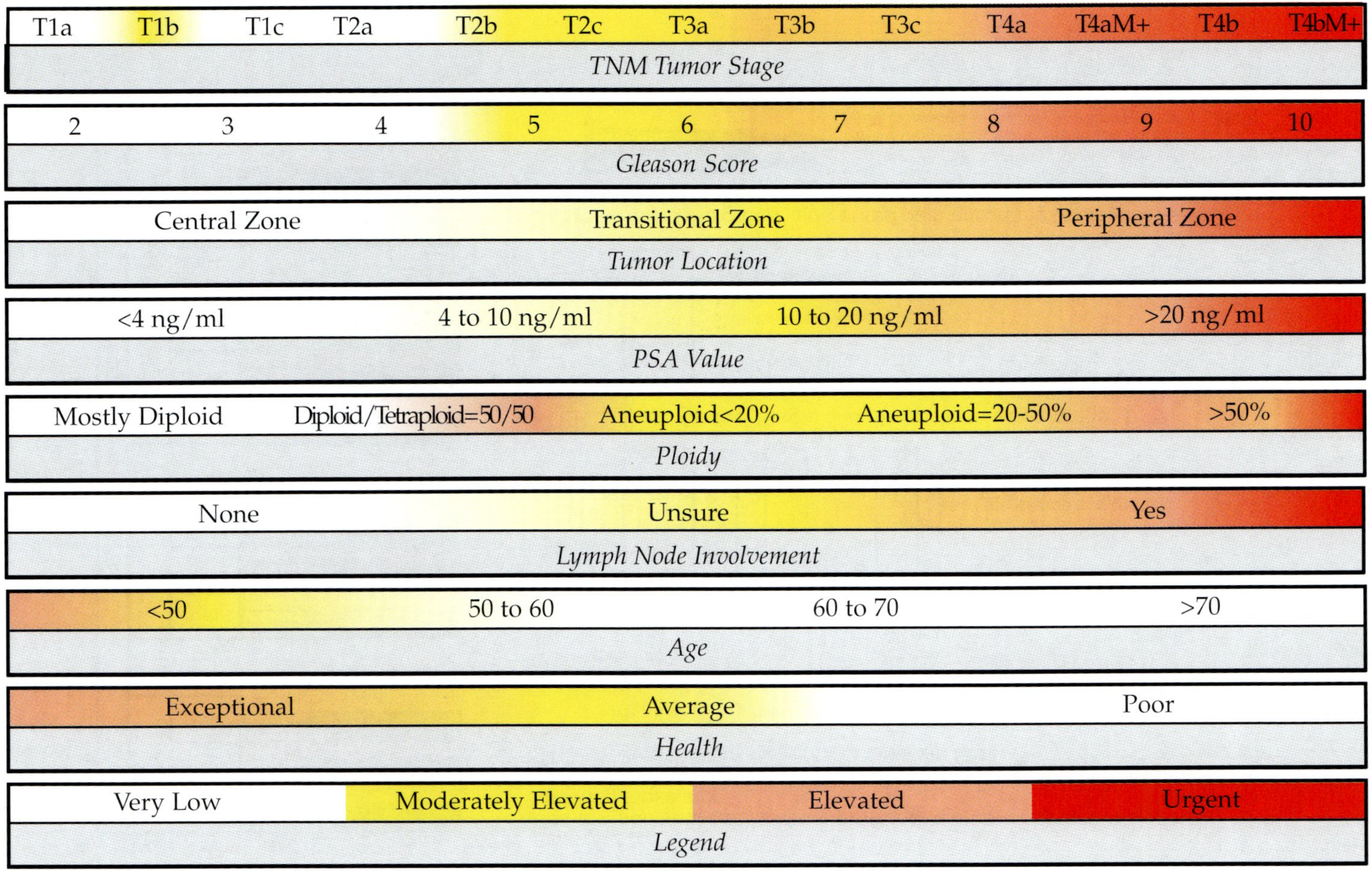

Figure 4
Treatment Decision Urgency

How to Use Treatment Options Charts

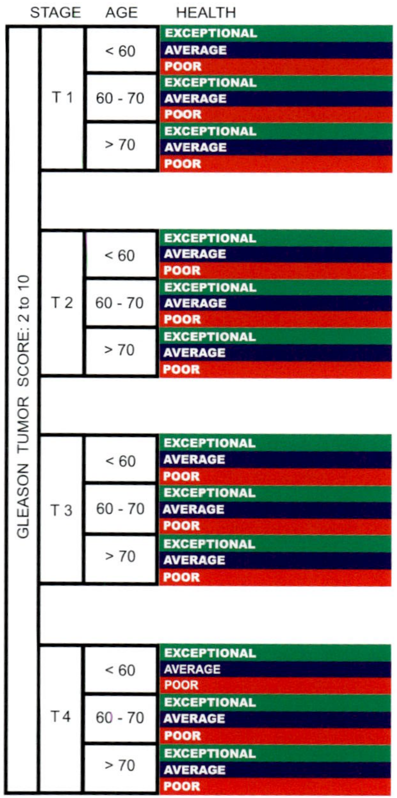

Use the indicated charts for determining appropriate treatment options, following these steps:

STEP 1. Find the chart for correct Gleason Score:

GLEASON TUMOR SCORE: 2 to 4 --- go to Figure 6
5 to 7 ------ go to Figure 7
8 to 10 -------- go to Figure 8

STEP 2. On the selected chart, first find Tumor Stage:

T 1 T 2 T 3 or T 4 as in the example at the left.

STEP 3. Then, for that Stage, find the applicable age-range:

< 60 Under sixty years

60 - 70 Sixty to seventy years

> 70 Over seventy years

STEP 4. Select the green, blue or red path according to state of health:

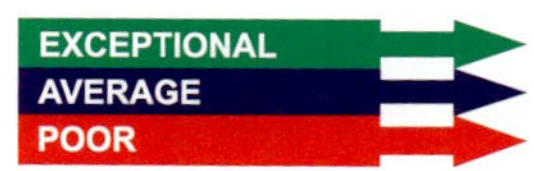

Follow the selected path (green, blue or red) to any white dot on that path. The arrow containing that dot points upward to identify a viable treatment option.

○ = Primary treatment option
□ = Co-partner for primary treatment
◇ = Secondary treatment

Figure 5
Instructional Chart for Finding Viable Treatment Options

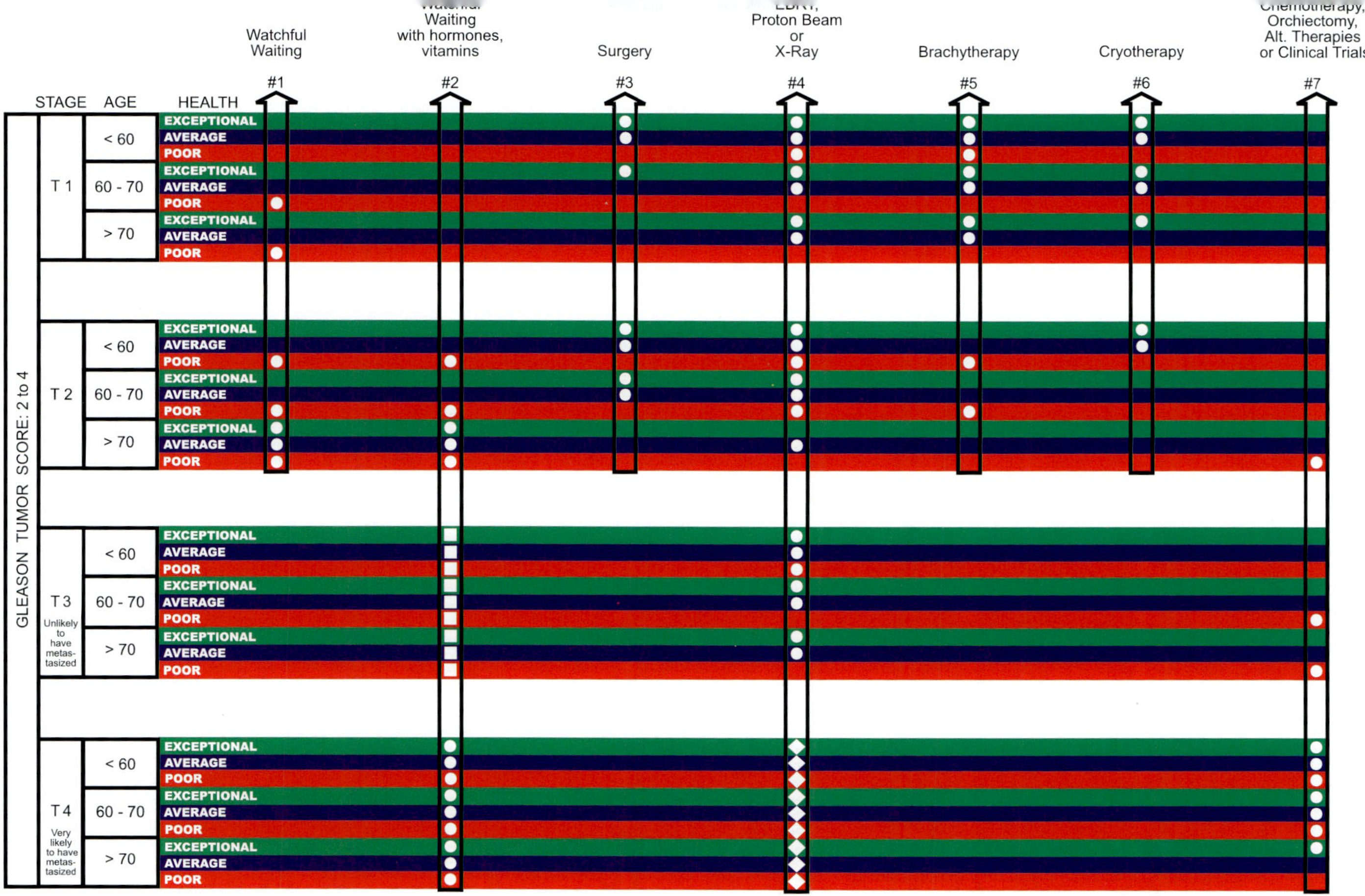

Figure 6
Treatment Options Chart: Gleason Score 2 to 4

○ = Primary treatment option
□ = Co-partner for primary treatment
◇ = Secondary treatment

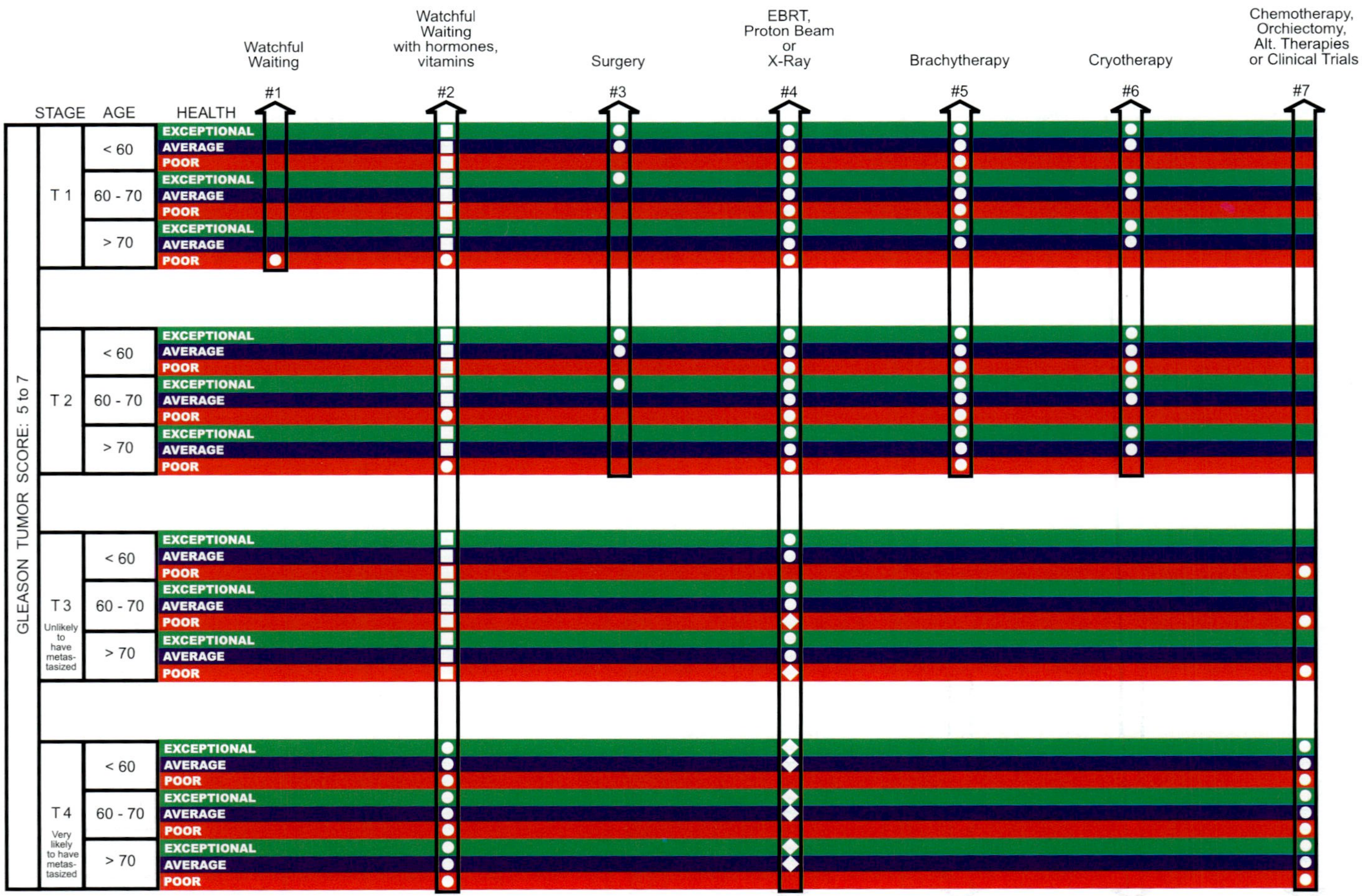

Figure 7
Treatment Options Chart: Gleason Score 5 to 7

○ = Primary treatment option
□ = Co-partner for primary treatment
◇ = Secondary treatment

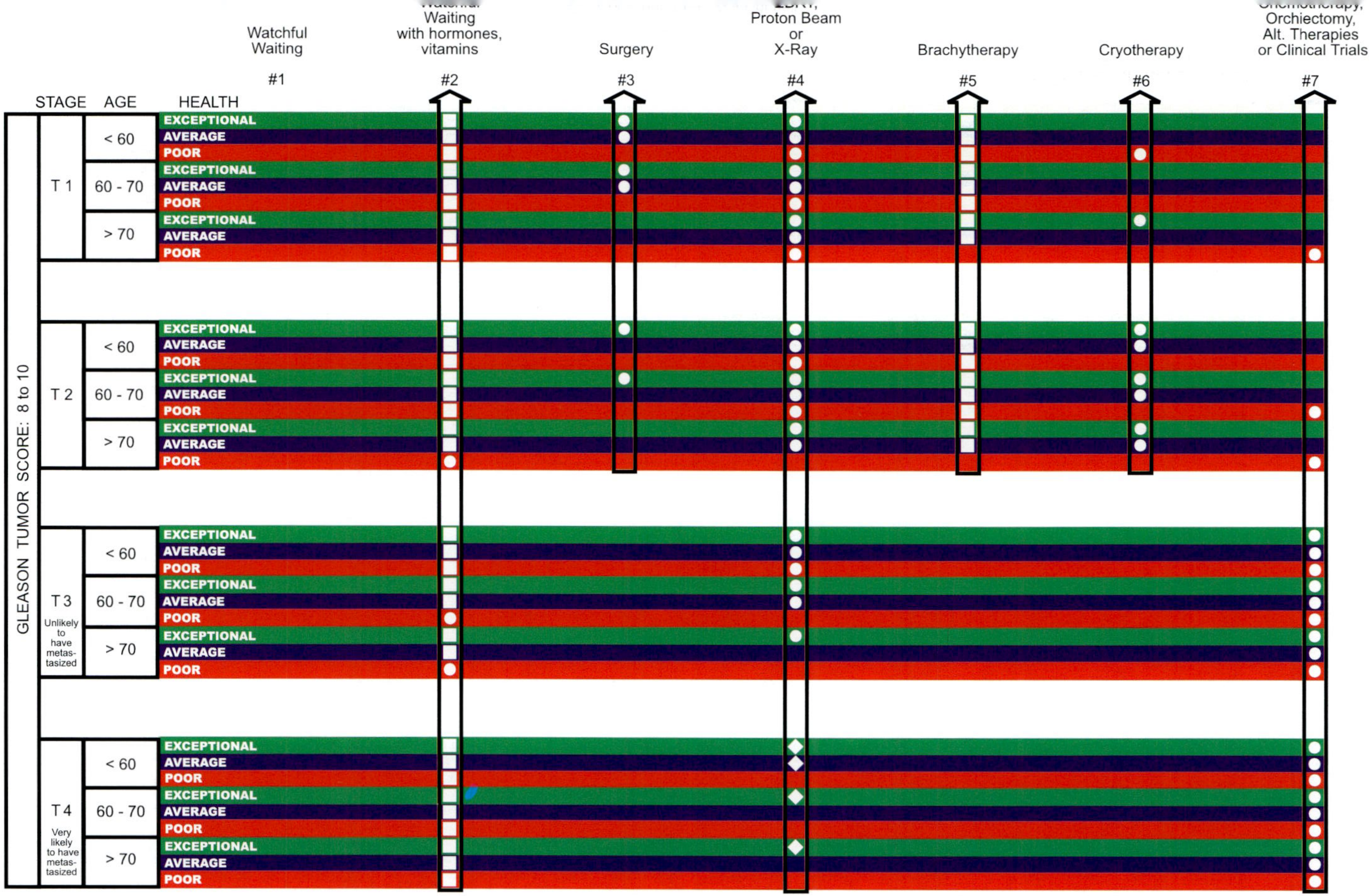

Figure 8
Treatment Options Chart: Gleason Score 8 to 10

○ = Primary treatment option
□ = Co-partner for primary treatment
◇ = Secondary treatment

PRIMARY TREATMENT	PRIMARY TREATMENT CLINICAL STATISTICS			FUTURE TREATMENT OPTIONS							
	Percent (1) Cases of Incontinence	Percent (1) Cases of Impotence	Recurrence Rate (2) 5 yr (upper) 10 yr (lower)	Watchful Waiting (#1)	Watchful Waiting with hormones (#2)	Surgery (#3)	EBRT: X-Ray only (#4a)	EBRT: X-Ray with Proton Beam or Brachytherapy (#4b)	Brachy-therapy (#5)	Cryotherapy (#6)	Chemotherapy, Orchiectomy, Alt. Therapies, Clinical Trials (#7)
Watchful Waiting (#1)	(Does not apply)			all future options open							
Watchful Waiting with hormones (#2)	(Does not apply)			all future options open							
Surgery (#3)	< 10%	30 - 50%	20 - 30% > 30%	OPEN	OPEN	CLOSED	OPEN	OPEN	OPEN	OPEN	OPEN
EBRT: X-Ray only (#4a)	< 10%	25 - 40%	5 - 20% 40 - 50%	OPEN	OPEN	Compromised	CLOSED	CLOSED	OPEN	Compromised	OPEN
EBRT: X-Ray with Proton Beam or Brachytherapy (#4b)	< 1%	20 - 40%	5 - 20% < 30%	OPEN	OPEN	Compromised	CLOSED	CLOSED	OPEN	Compromised	OPEN
Brachytherapy (#5)	< 2%	< 25%	5 - 10% 10 - 30%	OPEN	OPEN	Compromised	OPEN	Compromised	OPEN	OPEN	OPEN
Cryotherapy (#6)	< 5%	50 - 70%	15 - 20% (N/A)	OPEN	OPEN	Compromised	OPEN	OPEN	OPEN	OPEN	OPEN
Chemotherapy, Orchiectomy, Alt. Therapies or Clinical Trials (#7)	(Results are unpredictable and future options are unproven.)										

Figure 9
Future Treatment Options Chart

(1) Variations depend upon condition of health prior to treatment.

(2) Variations depend in large part on initial Gleason Score and Stage Value.

Gleason Score	Clinical Stage						
	T1a	T1b	T1c	T2a	T2b	T2c	T3a
				PSA 0.0 - 4.0 ng/ml			
2-4	100	85	92	88	76	82	-
5	100	78	91	81	67	73	-
6	100	68	69	72	54	60	42
7	-	54	55	61	41	46	-
8-10	-	-	-	48	31	-	-
				PSA 4.1- 10.0 ng/ml			
2-4	100	78	82	83	67	71	-
5	100	70	71	73	56	64	43
6	100	53	59	62	44	48	33
7	100	39	43	51	32	37	26
8-10	-	32	31	39	22	25	12
				PSA 10.1- 20.0 ng/ml			
2-4	100	-	-	61	52	-	-
5	100	49	55	58	43	37	26
6	-	36	41	44	28	37	19
7	-	24	24	36	19	24	14
8-10	-	11	-	29	14	15	9
				PSA > 20 ng/ml			
2-4	-	-	33	20	7	-	-
5	-	-	24	32	-	3	-
6	-	-	22	14	11	4	5
7	-	-	7	18	4	5	3
8-10	-	-	3	3	1	2	2

Figure 10-1 **Nomogram for predicting final pathological stage: Organ confined tumor.**

Gleason Score	Clinical Stage						
	T1a	T1b	T1c	T2a	T2b	T2c	T3a
				PSA 0.0 - 4.0 ng/ml			
2-4	0	15	22	14	26	17	-
5	0	22	30	20	43	26	-
6	0	30	34	29	46	38	59
7	-	43	40	39	59	50	-
8-10	-	-	-	50	68	-	-
				PSA 4.1- 10.0 ng/ml			
2-4	0	22	29	19	34	27	-
5	0	29	34	28	45	34	58
6	0	45	38	38	56	49	68
7	0	58	44	49	68	59	75
8-10	-	64	48	59	77	71	87
				PSA 10.1- 20.0 ng/ml			
2-4	0	-	-	40	49	-	-
5	0	49	40	43	58	61	75
6	-	62	45	56	73	59	82
7	-	73	52	64	81	73	86
8-10	-	87	-	70	86	82	92
				PSA > 20 ng/ml			
2-4	-	-	50	80	94	-	-
5	-	-	54	68	-	97	-
6	-	-	53	86	90	96	95
7	-	-	67	80	96	95	98
8-10	-	-	74	97	99	97	98

Figure 10-2 **Nomogram for predicting final pathological stage: Capsular penetration by tumor.**

Partin Nomogram Predictions of Pathological Stage

Gleason Score	Clinical Stage						
	T1a	T1b	T1c	T2a	T2b	T2c	T3a
				PSA 0.0 - 4.0 ng/ml			
2-4	0	1	< 1	1	2	2	-
5	0	3	< 1	2	4	4	-
6	0	6	1	5	9	9	8
–7	-	12	5	9	17	17	-
8-10	-	-	23	17	29	-	-
				PSA 4.1- 10.0 ng/ml			
2-4	0	2	< 1	1	3	3	-
5	0	4	< 1	3	6	6	5
6	0	9	1	6	11	12	11
7	0	18	5	12	22	23	18
8-10	-	29	23	22	38	40	40
				PSA 10.1- 20.0 ng/ml			
2-4	0	-	-	3	4	-	-
5	0	7	< 1	5	8	12	11
6	-	15	1	11	19	17	18
7	-	28	6	19	33	33	31
8-10	-	55	-	29	50	53	49
				PSA > 20 ng/ml			
2-4	-	-	< 1	12	30	-	-
5	-	-	< 1	11	-	29	-
6	-	-	2	35	40	53	31
7	-	-	9	31	73	62	55
8-10	-	-	31	81	93	73	65

Figure 10-3 **Nomogram for predicting final pathological stage: Seminal vesicle involvement by tumor.**

Gleason Score	Clinical Stage						
	T1a	T1b	T1c	T2a	T2b	T2c	T3a
				PSA 0.0 - 4.0 ng/ml			
2-4	0	2	< 1	1	2	4	-
5	0	4	1	2	4	9	-
6	0	8	2	3	9	17	15
7	-	15	2	7	18	31	-
8-10	-	-.	-	13	32	-	-
				PSA 4.1- 10.0 ng/ml			
2-4	0	2	1	1	2	5	-
5	0	4	1	2	5	10	8
6	0	9	2	4	11	19	16
7	0	18	3	8	20	34	28
8-10	-	30	5	15	35	53	50
				PSA 10.1- 20.0 ng/ml			
2-4	0	-	-	1	3	-	-
5	0	5	3	2	6	13	11
6	-	11	4	5	13	22	20
7	-	21	7	9	24	39	35
8-10	-	41	-	17	40	59	54
				PSA > 20 ng/ml			
2-4	-	-	6	2	7	-	-
5	-	-	9	3	-	29	-
6	-	-	8	9	18	53	31
7	-	-	24	11	44	62	55
8-10	-	-	41	35	76	73	65

Figure 10-4 **Nomogram for predicting final pathological stage: Lymph node involvement.**

Partin Nomogram Predictions of Pathological Stage

for a second therapy may result in greater incontinence or impotence, or it may not be as effective a treatment the second time around. For instance, if cryotherapy is used as a secondary treatment after previous radiation, the chance of incontinence increases to approximately 50 percent.

All of these clinical factors are more favorable for patients who are relatively young and in full health. As we age, and as our health deteriorates, we can expect less optimistic clinical statistics.

All these things ought to be considered while you are deciding on your primary treatment. The charts and tables in the guide include all the factors that define you as a particular patient: Gleason score, tumor stage, PSA, age and health. The clinical statistics and the considerations regarding future treatment options relate to your emotional makeup and what you are comfortable with. The combination of all these considerations will guide you to your particular treatment decision.

The statistics for incontinence, impotence, and recurrence are rough estimates made from a number of sources. Since they have been derived from the major clinics the numbers are as optimistic as you can expect. While not precise, they do indicate the relative differences among various treatments that you ought to consider in your decision-making. It is likely that if you experienced problems with bladder control or had erectile dysfunction prior to treatment, your chance of having these side effects increases. A person who has never had incontinence or impotence problems may be somewhat less likely to suffer severe side effects in the future.

If this chapter has been a bit difficult to absorb, don't give up. Chapters 15 and 16 take you step-by-step through the option charts for several different cases. You will see how a treatment decision for my situation and for several others can be determined.

Remember This

It is difficult to arrive at the best treatment decision. Even physicians in the field disagree. But, most do agree that the correct Gleason score and stage determination, and whether or not the tumor is still confined within the prostate, are the most important treatment choice determinants.

In Chapter 23 you will learn about techniques that produce images of your prostate and tumor. Soon, these techniques will be used to integrate many aspects of each man's condition. The day may come when these techniques will allow us to custom-make treatments for each individual patient.

The Treatment Option Charts are an attempt to display the choices before you in a visual but scientific manner. The Future Treatment Option Chart is important to you and directly affects your future quality of life. A careful study of all the charts, and discussions of them with your physicians, ought to give you confidence as you approach your treatment.

Chapter 10

Watchful Waiting

Watchful waiting is a "therapy" wherein nothing is done by way of invasive treatments. Radiation, the surgeon's knife, or extreme chemical treatments do not play a part in this approach. On the surface, this is a curious avenue to follow for successful treatment of prostate cancer. In Europe this therapy is more common than it is in the United States. Indeed, there are historical statistical data from European countries that show that the life expectancy for some cancer patients who opt for watchful waiting is just as high as it is for patients who undergo surgery or radiation. The situation is actively debated in medical circles, however.

Older medical literature indicates that radiation and surgical therapies do not provide an improved quality of life for more than a year or so beyond what would occur by doing nothing. This is part of the argument against active PSA screenings of the population.

But Dr. Fernand Labrie, of the Centre de Recherche du Centre Hospitalier de L'Universite Laval, in Quebec, believes that while prostate cancer does progress slowly, it inevitably leads to distant metastases and death if left untreated and sufficient time elapses. Thus, one has to conclude that deferred treatment of any kind is inadvisable for any man in otherwise good health who has more than a decade of life left to him.

In the United States, we prefer a more pro-active approach to prostate cancer. But, depending upon stage, grade, health and age of a patient, watchful waiting could be a sensible option.

As outlined in the Treatment Option Charts, there are perfectly good reasons to select watchful waiting as an intelligent treatment. If you are aged or in poor health, your physician can predict from his actuarial tables that you will die of other causes before your cancer can disrupt and threaten your quality of life. As an example, if you are over age 75, in poor health and have a low Gleason grade, well-differentiated cancer, staged at T1, you can be "reassured" that you do not have time enough to allow this cancer to progress and threaten you. You will be one of us who will die with cancer, rather than from cancer. In this case your longevity and quality of life will not benefit from surgery or radiation therapies. Indeed, your quality of life will be degraded by these more aggressive therapies. There is no reason to undergo the trauma of, say, surgery. You do not need to be "cured" of cancer. You can live with it as a very slowly progressing "chronic" condition.

This is also true if your Gleason score is below 6 and your PSA doubling time is more than five years. The doubling time shows that this is not an aggressive tumor. If, however, you have a higher Gleason score and a rapid PSA doubling time, you are in danger. Tumors of Gleason score 7 or above are the only ones that can change from being confined within the prostate to causing death in a short time. Watchful waiting for this situation is not an appropriate treatment, even if you are older than 75.

The most promising patient for watchful waiting treatment is over 70 years and has a low Gleason grade tumor that is not palpable on the DRE, meaning that it is staged very low. PSA doubling time should be low. If you choose this therapy, you will have little or no change in your present quality of life. You will most likely die of other causes before the cancer has a chance to overtake you.

Watchful waiting can also be viewed as a kind of bet, a bet that new treatment techniques will soon be available. There are a number of research studies that promise a chemical, DNA, or cancer-blocking technique to combat tumor growth. Currently, this is not a sure bet, but progress is being made in this field.

The choice to follow a watchful waiting path must, I believe, be discussed in detail with your physician. Both of you must be comfortable with this decision and with any combined treatments, such as hormone therapy, as well as with the methods of monitoring your prostate during your watchful waiting. Monitoring must be done because you do run a risk if you make this choice using wrong assumptions (or have an understaged condition), or do not maintain a very close watch on your progress. If you are not careful, you may wind up forced to deal with an advanced case of cancer. You run the risk that at some point the window of opportunity for a complete cure will close on you.

Your discussions with your physicians must take into account your basic clinical numbers, PSA, Gleason grade, and stage. Your age, general health situation, and personal preference will be the important factors in such a decision. In all these discussions, make sure you keep in mind the conditions or changes that would require a more aggressive treatment for you. Obviously regular PSA and DRE testing must be a routine part of your life. As insignificant as your numbers may seem now, your condition should not be ignored!

With watchful waiting, you will not experience any hospitalization or disruption to your life style, other than regular visits to your physician.

Remember This

In America we are too pro-active to employ watchful waiting, unless the patient has a very low Gleason score, is elderly, or in poor health. If these conditions do not describe you, do not listen to physicians who recommend doing nothing to treat your condition. Your life depends upon a correct treatment decision that is appropriate for your clinical condition, age, and health.

Watchful waiting, with or without hormone use, can be combined with a prescribed diet. For appropriate patients, some physicians may employ such treatments so long as

pre-determined PSA and tumor monitoring schedules are maintained.

Chapter 11

Watchful Waiting with Hormones

Many physicians use a watchful waiting approach for cancer patients, but combine this with treatments of partial or total hormone blockage. The blockage of testosterone from the testes and two androgens from the adrenal glands can be achieved with the use of various androgen-suppressing drugs, some injected and some taken orally. Often these two methods are used together.

If a man is older than 70 years, has a Gleason score of 6 or less, and a life expectancy of 10 years or less, he might reasonably decide on watchful waiting coupled with combined hormone therapy.

This approach also can work for elderly men who have advanced cancer where tumor material has escaped the prostate and has invaded tissues that surround the prostate. These patients can not be treated successfully by surgery and perhaps not by radiation. Thus T3 and T4 staged patients can be helped, but not cured, by this approach. In this case, the goal is palliative for a gradually worsening condition and cannot be thought of as curative. Unless the patient is in very poor health, some type of intervention ought to be used, perhaps radiation of some kind. At least the primary tumor could be brought under control, and this may help the hormone treatment control the secondary tumors.

With *intermittent* hormone therapy, the patient receives the hormone blockage drugs until his PSA value reaches a "nadir point" at a very low level. Medicines are then stopped and the PSA value is watched until it rises to 10 ng/ml or perhaps 20 ng/ml. At this point the medicines are resumed and used until the PSA value falls again to a low level. This cycling is more effective in allowing the patient a decent quality of life than would be the case with constant hormone blockage treatment. Typically, life can be extended by this treatment for more than three years, and many physicians claim success in keeping their patients alive for a decade or more.

Tumors with Gleason scores greater than 7 will probably be less controllable with hormonal therapy than less aggressive tumors will be.

If you intend to be treated by this method, you will not require hospitalization, but you will need a monthly or quarterly hormone injection from your doctor or local hospital. You will also have to maintain a regular daily routine to take oral hormones. You will have hot flashes and perhaps some general weakness and weight change, and will require more rest than you are used to. Your interest in sex will lessen. Some physicians do not advocate hormone use. These arguments are outlined in Chapter 17.

It should be noted that prolonged use of hormones can bring about a "chemical castration," where the testes are so damaged that they are unable to recover and to produce testosterone even after the hormone blockage is stopped. Your doctor will determine how long it is "safe" for you to take the hormones.

Remember This

Combined hormonal therapies (CHT) will slow or halt tumor growth, at least for some period of time. CHT, if used indefinitely, loses its effectiveness in most cases. If it is used for more than, say, a year, as a *preparation* for surgery or radiation, the therapy itself could ultimately bring about chemical castration. Thus, it may cause the very impotence one is trying to avoid by using hormones instead of surgery or radiation treatments. Thus, this treatment should be employed judiciously. A younger man might use this treatment in conjunction with surgery or radiation. To an elderly man, who may no longer be sexually active, impotence may not be a serious objection.

Chapter 12

Surgery

Every year some 100,000 surgeries are performed in the United States for removal of a cancerous prostate. There are a number of things you need to know about surgery, the most common primary treatment for prostate cancer:

1. It is the oldest method of treatment and so has the most long term survival and morbidity data from which to make outcome predictions. Surgical techniques are used in more than 50 percent of all prostate cancer treatments. Some surgeons will use this fact as argument against newer techniques such as proton beam or seed implantation therapies. Neither seed implantation nor proton beam therapy has extensive ten-year survival data, let alone the 15-year to 20-year statistical record that the surgeon can show you.

Do not be overly influenced by surgery's history and data.

The statistical data reported for radical prostatectomies are flawed. This is because the reported data do not include results achieved by the thousands of surgeons not associated with the major clinics specializing in this surgery. If these data were included in the numbers we see in the literature, the statistics would be far less encouraging.

2. If your cancer is truly located within the prostate, surgery has an excellent chance of completely removing cancer, unless cancer cells are spread via blood and lymph during a poorly executed surgery. If you have a tumor that has *escaped* from the prostate capsule, surgery rarely cures. Other therapies, particularly radiation of some kind, will be necessary. Surgery has a relatively high risk of incontinence and impotence. These side effects are more prevalent in men older than 70.

3. There are two basic kinds of surgery; radical prostatectomy (the older type of procedure), and nerve-sparing prostatectomy, a procedure specifically designed to spare the potency nerves and developed by Dr. Patrick Walsh at John Hopkins Hospital in Baltimore. The book by Dr. Marc

Garnick, listed in the bibliography, will give you details of what to expect from either type of surgery.

4. If you are staged T3 or above, then the implication is that cancer cells have spread outside the prostate capsule. In this event, surgical removal of the prostate will not be successful for you. Surgery is not advised, unless your physicians (note I use the plural, as a radiologist is now required on your team) think it is advisable to remove the prostate as the primary source of tumor activity. It may be that once it is removed, the radiologist, who will be required to find and radiate cancerous tissue outside the prostate, will be more effective in doing so. However, this is a debated issue in the field. Some physicians do not believe in removing the prostate in this circumstance. They prefer to treat it systemically with hormone therapy or with more aggressive chemotherapy.

Remember the comments about under-staging of your condition. Prostate cancer that is not truly confined to the prostate has a high incidence of recurrence. Patients whose cancer has spread beyond the prostate will not be cured by surgery alone. Usually surgical patients require future radiation in order to kill any tumor tissue left behind after the surgery.

5. Surgery has one important advantage: It does not close any doors for future therapy in the event of a recurrence. In the event that cancer was not fully removed by surgery, you still have all the options of radiation, cryosurgery, hormone treatments, etc., left to employ.

6. The *location* within the prostate of an "organ confined" tumor may rule out surgery. For instance, if the tumor is too close to the bladder sphincter, you and your urologist might decide on radiation in order to minimize a potential future problem with incontinence. Most men develop tumors in the apex region of the prostate.

Let's take the three basic numbers of your condition

(PSA, Gleason score, and tumor stage value) and look at some historical data that have been compiled from 1,186 cases of radical surgery performed between 1985 and 1995 at Johns Hopkins University of Medicine. Figure 10 shows what the *pathological* condition really was for these men, relating back to the original *clinical* assessment with PSA, Gleason score, and stage. This is a very important tradeoff nomogram that you should study in detail. (A nomogram is a visual device used to display complicated relationships among various kinds of data). These tables are now widely recognized in the profession and are relied upon for proper patient management. Figure 10 is taken from an article titled "The Use of Prostate Specific Antigen, Clinical Stage and Gleason Score to Predict Pathological Stage in Men with Localized Prostate Cancer," *The Journal of Urology,* volume 150, 1993, pp. 172-173 by Partin, et al. It is widely cited in the literature. The numbers in these tables are probabilities shown as percent. They show the probability that you actually have disease totally confined within the prostate (Fig. 10-1,) or an extension beyond the prostate capsule (Fig. 10-2,) or further invasion to the seminal vesicles (Fig. 10-3,) or spread to the lymph nodes (Fig. 10-4.) Early in my investigation, when one of my physicians showed me this study, I took the first step toward my real-world education. It was a very sobering experience for me. In fact, it was a shock.

Now, it is pretty clear what decisions you need to make regarding surgery. If you are in the upper left corner of Figure 10-1, you have an almost assured success rate of removing cancer from your system if you choose a prostatectomy, assuming you are willing to accept the incontinence and impotence risk statistics that go with surgery, Figure 9.

But, if you are in the lower right corner of Partin's table, your chances of eliminating your cancer with surgery are very poor. For instance, if you are a Gleason score 8, with a T3 condition and a really elevated PSA, your chances of success with surgical removal are only 2 percent, as shown in Figure 10-1.

There are two other conclusions one could reach when reviewing these data, which were obtained from actual documented surgical histories. You will recall that a T1 or T2 staging means *by definition* that the cancer has not escaped the prostate nor spread to other sites in the body. Note the statistics in Partin's table for the mid range of conditions, say a T2b, Gleason score 6 and a PSA of 10 ng/ml. This says that the success rate for surgery in this category is only 44 percent, success being defined as a zero PSA level after surgery.

There is a contradiction here. If surgery completely removes a cancerous prostate where escape has *not* occurred (a T1 or T2 stage), how is it possible that only 44 percent of patients are cancer free after surgery? I can think of two possibilities:

1. The original clinical staging estimate was incorrect. That is, the condition was originally underestimated and the tumor had actually spread farther than originally thought.
2. Cancer cells were spread to the blood or other body fluids *during* the operation to remove the prostate. As infrequently as this may happen, it is a real risk. Often, examinations of the fluids removed during surgery show free cancer cells in them.

These facts may explain why almost half of the men who have had radical prostatectomies require additional treatment within five years of surgery. This is very sobering, and is rarely discussed with prospective patients.

Either way, this chart causes second thoughts for the majority of us who find ourselves in the middle ground on the table. If you are in the upper left of the table and are elderly, you can almost forget about cancer as a threat to your life. If you are in the lower right side of the table, you would be wise to consider other means (quickly) to solve your specific condition, as it is certain that surgery will not cure. Radiation is a powerful alternative to surgery in this situation, although a case can be made for prostatectomy just to remove the original source of the cancer, despite some arguments against this. Understand that you will *also* need radiation to cover the entire area of the prostate bed into which cancer cells most likely have spread. Radiation here is the primary treatment, while any surgery acts as the secondary assist procedure.

Surgery will require major alterations to your normal routine. This treatment is a major event which will take a toll on your body and will require considerable time for recovery. You will spend at least one week in the hospital, and will need four to six weeks of recovery time at home. You will be on a catheter for most of your recovery time. Plan on losing two full months of work if you choose surgery. After surgery you will need time to regain your strength to normal levels. You will need some time to regain full bladder control. All these considerations have to be weighed regarding your work and travel routines.

Remember This

If you have decided on surgery, join your local prostate cancer support group first and conduct your private survey. Find out which local surgeons gave the best morbidity statistics to your fellow members. Trust the experiences of your fellow patients, rather than taking any physician's counsel at face value. Compare their statistics with those produced by the major American clinics and published in the literature. Then compare your physician's statistics with what you have learned.

We see only data published by the big specialist centers and none from the small practitioner. If we could somehow factor in these unknown statistics, the published morbidity

and mortality rates for surgery would be more unattractive than they are.

Chapter 13

Radiation

Every year in the United States about 100,000 men undergo radiation treatment for prostate cancer. Radiation of one kind or another can be effective in curing cancer. It may not be as effective for early stage, confined tumors, as cleanly performed surgery is (although there are now data that suggest that it may be just as effective), but it is a viable treatment for men with localized tumors or with tumors that have reached the prostate margins. Radiation, if it does not actually kill all tumor cells, may cause those that remain to grow so slowly after treatment that cancer will never cause you a problem during the remainder of your life. Many physicians believe that in some cases radiation "stuns" the cancer and renders it inactive. Tumor cells cannot repair damage caused by radiation as well as normal cells can.

Radiation is a good treatment for elderly men who may be at risk in a surgical procedure, or for men who, as a matter of personal preference, do not wish to consider surgery. Radiation of any kind may cause incontinence or impotence, but usually these risks are lower for radiation than for surgery.

Four important things you need to know about radiation treatments are:

Types of radiation treatment
Total **allowed dosage**
Loss of **pathological stage assessment**
Future treatment compromises

1. Types of Radiation Treatment

There are several kinds of radiation treatments that you can choose from. In the past, there was only old-fashioned pelvic area external beam X-ray radiation, but now there are improved X-ray treatments and other effective radiation methods to kill cancer tumors. These new technologies are replacing the older methods, and you are advised to insist on them if you choose radiation therapy.

The main challenge for the oncologist is to determine what type of radiation is most appropriate for your particular condition. Can you successfully be treated by radioactive seeds alone, or is a combination of seeds with 3D conformal external beam radiation best?

Radiation techniques may be summarized as follows:

External Beam General Area Radiation:

Standard pelvic area X-ray radiation, with limited focussing of the beams, covers a wide area of your pelvis. This treatment option is the old stand-by radiation method that has been used for decades. The books listed in the bibliography will cover details of this method. Since this method of radiation is being superseded rapidly by more modern radiation treatments, most up-to-date radiologists do not recommend it. Many feel the new 3D conformal focussed external beam or seed implantation radiation technologies will completely replace the older radiation methods in a few of years.

3D Conformal External Beam Radiation:

Three-dimensional conformal X-ray radiation aims radiation from many directions, or "poles" of attack. That is why this technology is called a three-dimensional "conformal" radiation treatment. With the aid of computer studies of your prostate, the radiation beams are directed *precisely* to the volume of the prostate, with added emphasis on the area where your tumor is known to be located. In conformal radiation treatments, damage to surrounding healthy tissue is minimized.

Proton External Beam Radiation:

Proton beam radiation uses large *nuclear* particles rather than X-rays. Proton beam radiation is often applied in combination with standard conformal X-ray radiation therapy. Since the proton beam is made up of nuclear particles rather than high energy photons or X-rays, it can deliver energetic radiation to the prostate with minimal damage to the normal tissue that the beam must travel through when entering and leaving the pelvis. If this treatment is chosen, the conformal X-ray radiation portion of the treatment is often of lesser strength than if X-ray radiation alone were to be used, thus lessening the morbidity effects from this source of treatment.

The two major centers in America that offer proton beam radiation are Loma Linda University Medical Center in Loma Linda, California, and Massachusetts General Hospital in Boston.

Brachytherapy (Radioactive Seed Implantation):

Brachytherapy brings powerful radiation directly into the prostate and to the tumor site. Tiny metal pellets (called "seeds") containing a radioactive substance are injected into the prostate. Many years ago brachytherapy (common names are seed implantation and interstitial radiation) was attempted, but since the radioactive seeds were rather primitive and there was poor placement accuracy for the surgeon in directing the seeds into the prostate, the procedure fell into disuse, and wisely so. With the advent of computer-assisted sonogram monitoring and far more accurate seed manufacture and emplacement equipment, brachytherapy is becoming a recognized and effective method of treatment. Because the accuracy of seed implantation is so precise, the treatment minimizes damage to healthy nearby tissue. Many clinics now employ this method exclusively with excellent results.

Brachy means "short distance," indicating that the radiation emitted from the seeds extends only a very short distance, so the seeds can deliver a very powerful radiation dose directly to the prostate and tumor with minimal exposure to healthy tissues surrounding the prostate. The advantage of seed implantation is that the volume of intense radioactivity is approximately one half inch in diameter. Thus, this method of treatment can deliver twice as much radiation to the tumor as is possible with external beam radiation therapy. In this case, the radioactivity source is in almost direct contact with the tumor cells, in contrast to external beam radiation which originates from outside the body.

The radioactivity of the seeds also has a short duration of time. The "half-life" of palladium-103 seeds is about two weeks, while the half-life of iodine-125 seeds is longer, about 60 days. In the case of palladium seeds, this means that in two weeks the radiation dose has dropped to one half the original dose, and two weeks later it will be one half what it was after the first two weeks. In six to eight weeks the radiation level will be negligible. There is no risk in carrying the seeds with you for the rest of your life. And, no, you will not set off airport security alarm systems!

Brachytherapy is a reasonable choice of treatment if one wishes to avoid surgery or standard X-ray radiation. Seed implantation, however, is often combined with a course of external X-ray radiation if the tumor has reached the prostate capsule wall or if there is suspicion that cancer cells have escaped into the area surrounding the prostate. But, as with proton beam therapy, the seeds concentrate radiation within the prostate, and the external beam radiation dosage can be lower than when it is used as the sole source of radiation.

For aggressive tumors, Gleason score 7 or higher, implantation alone is not advised. These tumors require additional radiation to be fully eradicated. In this case, brachytherapy should be used as a co-partner therapy, with EBRT as the primary treatment.

There are three main types of brachytherapy, and these can be combined with external beam radiation in various ways, depending on the particular factors of each patient.

Radioactive seeds alone:
- Iodine seeds for lower grade tumor conditions.
- Palladium seeds for higher grade tumor conditions.

External Beam radiation combined with seeds:
- Combined with iodine seeds.
- Combined with palladium seeds.

Temporarily implanted seeds of very high potency.

The book by Kaltenbach, listed in the bibliography, gives a fine personal account of a man who selected seed implantation therapy. The Fortune magazine article by Intel's Andy Grove shows the course that Grove traveled to reach the high density radiation treatment solution.

2. Total Radiation Dosage

Your body can withstand only so much radiation over your lifetime. This means if you choose radiation, you have limits to the amount of radiation you can use later if the first treatment fails to eradicate your cancer.

External beam radiation treatments are given in small-dose amounts daily over a period of five or six weeks. This is because the non-cancerous cells that will also be radiated will be able to recover each day from the effects of the radiation, while the cancerous cells will not. By spreading out the treatment time the radiation will have a minimal effect on normal cells close to your prostate.

Basically, you can use radiation *only once* if you choose external beam X-ray radiation applied at the fullest dosage. But, if you choose proton beam radiation, or if you use a lower external beam dosage, you may still have the option of brachytherapy if you need it later. Similarly, if a primary treatment with brachytherapy fails, you may be able to use proton beam therapy or a limited dose X-ray treatment. And, you can also have a second limited implantation of seeds.

3. Loss of Pathological Stage Assessment

One disadvantage of radiation treatments is that there is no way to find out the actual pathological stage value. Surgery discovers this at the time of the operation. However, if your PSA value begins to rise after radiation, then it is possible, via a surgical lymphadenectomy, to obtain biopsy material from your lymph nodes to determine if the cancer has spread. Also, the new multispectral MRI scans are very accurate in revealing whether or not your tumor has escaped the prostate walls and whether or not any tumor material remains after your primary treatment.

4. Future Treatment Compromises

Radiation, whether X-ray or seed radiation, compromises the option for future surgery if radiation fails as your primary treatment. Only a few very specialized surgeons are willing to remove a prostate filled with tiny seeds of spent radioactive material. Furthermore, in the case of external beam radiation, the prostate is converted from pliable tissue into hardened scar tissue. I am overstating the case here on purpose. Surgery *can* be performed, but it is far more difficult for the surgeon than if surgery had been used as a primary treatment method. If surgery is done *after* radiation, you stand a far greater chance of downside morbidity, such as increased incontinence or serious impairment to the nerves that control potency. There are, however, surgeons who specialize in what is called "salvage surgery" if this is required.

The choice of radiation of some kind may depend upon

your age and health. Although, at first glance, surgery may show better long-term results, radiation is perfectly sensible as a primary choice, especially for older men. Total eradication for the long term may not be as important as it would be for a younger man. Mere control of tumor growth is a valid decision in this case.

One side benefit of radiation is that you probably will not experience difficulties in the future from benign prostatic hypertrophy (BPH).

External beam or proton beam radiation treatments will not take the toll on your body that surgery does. Most likely you will not experience physical reactions from your treatments, although some men may develop low grade RTOG symptoms or general tiredness. Some men need a recovery period to regain full bladder control. Radiation treatments take time. You will need up to six weeks of *daily* trips to the hospital. If the clinic is not near your home you will need to calculate travel and lodging expenses. Men who are treated in cities where they work will not need to alter their routines, other than to schedule the daily interruptions. Usually, the patient will spend an hour each day at the radiation clinic.

Brachytherapy treatment is a greater intrusion of your body and disruption of your routine than are external beam treatments. No matter what you are told about the ease of these treatments, your body will respond to the intrusion and seed implantation. This procedure will take place in a surgical theater at a medical clinic. Most likely you will be an outpatient for this procedure. Some men have little or no immediate physical discomfort, while others require a catheter for several days because of swelling that constricts the urethra. You may be given local or general anesthesia. Usually, the implantation takes about an hour. Few men require overnight hospitalization.

Unless you experience difficulties urinating you will be able to return to your normal routine within a few days, although most likely you will find yourself visiting the bathroom more often than usual. And most likely you will get up several times during the night.

Remember This

You have a number of radiation treatments to choose from. Depending upon your unique critical factors, you should be able to determine whether or not radiation is the preferred treatment method, and which suits you best.

There are a number of secondary factors to compare among the various types of radiation.These are noted in Table 4. Discuss with your radiologist the secondary effects that each therapy could cause. The task before a radiation oncologist is to deliver a full lethal dose of radiation to the prostate and tumor, while minimizing damage to surrounding tissues and organs.

Although the newer 3D conformal beam radiation techniques do not yet have the long statistical history that surgery can muster, the five-year survival data are impressive. The five-year survival number for patients with high grade prostate cancer treated with surgery shows no advantage over those treated with radiation. This gives added reassurance that radiation now competes effectively with surgery. Your radiologist may combine various radiation techniques, such as conformal beam with seed implantation or a combination of proton beam radiation with conformal beam radiation. He will also advise you to stop all antioxidant medications such as vitamins C and E so tumor cells are rendered vulnerable to radiation.

Advocates of the newer radiation techniques believe that the days of standard prostactectomy surgery are numbered. There are even prominent surgeons who agree with this prediction.

Chapter 14

Cryosurgery

Cryosurgery (or cryotherapy or cryoablation) has been around in one form or another for almost 50 years, but new technologies make it an improved procedure that is becoming more and more a treatment of choice.

The U.S. Government Health Care Financing Administration, after considerable study, has concluded that cryosurgery produces results comparable to external beam radiation and brachytherapy. They now recognize this as a valid treatment and will cover the treatment for Medicare patients.

In cryosurgery, delicate probes are inserted into the prostate and liquid nitrogen is injected under controlled conditions to freeze the prostate and the tumor material. A patient who undergoes cryosurgery will have less physical trauma and a faster recovery period than one who has a radical surgical removal of his prostate. Cryosurgery may be equivalent in effectiveness to brachytherapy for low-risk patients and may be superior for those who have a higher Gleason score or higher stage value.

Cryosurgery is a respectable and rational choice, and can be seriously considered because of recent advances in computer and sonogram technology. This technology allows the surgeon accurate control of the placement of the freezing probes. Most importantly, he can watch on his monitor, as the "freezing front" travels across the prostate, killing prostate and tumor tissue as it advances. The surgeon can stop the freezing front exactly where he wants to and not a millimeter farther.

As a technique competing with surgery, cryosurgery appears to have greater success for patients whose initial PSA is greater than 20 ng/ml. For patients between 10 ng/ml and 20 ng/ml, cryosurgery is 50 percent more effective in reducing PSA levels to near zero than is surgery.

There are a number of things you need to know about

this treatment option:

1. Cryosurgery can be applied a number of times if necessary. You do not close or compromise options for future use, as you do with radiation.

2. Properly done cryosurgery disrupts your life far less than a surgical procedure and has a minimal effect on your urinary tract. It does not require a general anesthesia and there is a minimal loss of blood. Compared to surgery it is far less traumatic to your body, and recovery is swift. It is a far less expensive therapy than surgery or radiation treatments. There is little or no incontinence with cryosurgery.

But, at least for the short term, it will render you completely impotent, because the nerves adjacent to your prostate will be frozen and damaged. If the surgeon is careful and the treatment proceeds routinely, you stand better than a 50-50 chance of potency returning after a year or so elapses and your nerve tissues begin to regenerate themselves to a healthier state. Compared to radical surgery, hospitalization time and recovery time are minimal. Poorly administered cryosurgery can result in a number of RTOG side effects (see Table 4, page 37) that can result in a poor quality of life for you.

3. Cryosurgery is a possible choice for men with stage T1 and T2 cancer, especially if they want to avoid the trauma of radical surgery, or if they are uncomfortable with the idea of radiation treatments. For an elderly man or a patient who is ill, this procedure holds significant advantages.

4. Cryosurgery's most important use may be its role as follow-up procedure in the event of failed primary treatments of any kind, or if a small patch of residual tumor material remains after radiation. The procedure has an impressive record in reducing PSA levels to near zero. It is far less invasive than salvage surgery following radiation treatments, although statistics show that cryosurgery after primary radiation treatment results in increased levels of

incontinence, approaching 50 percent. This fact may affect your decision to have radiation treatment as primary therapy.

Cryosurgery will have a physical effect on your body, but certainly less of an effect than surgery will. This procedure requires a full day's hospitalization as well as several days of recovery time. In addition, it requires a temporary external catheter tube to be inserted through your abdomen. This catheter has the formidable name "percutaneous suprapubic tube." Do not let this short-term inconvenience deter you if you are satisfied with the other treatment aspects of cryosurgery. You will have this for up to four weeks. It is removed as an outpatient procedure when your urine flow becomes strong enough. Eighty percent of cryosurgery patients who are sexually active prior to treatment regain their potency if they use either injection therapy or the vacuum pump. This statistic seems to improve after a year or so.

Remember This

We now have almost a decade of accumulated clinical data on this new technique, so cryosurgery is taking its place as a primary treatment option. Cryosurgery now offers serious competition to surgery as an effective treatment, especially for men who wish to avoid a radical prostatectomy or for men whose health cannot withstand the rigors of major surgery.

Cryosurgery has significant advantages as far as short-term morbidity trauma to the patient is concerned. It also costs less than surgery.

Cryosurgery is gaining credibility mostly as a salvage technique when primary surgery or radiation therapy has failed. With each passing year, the techniques and clinical

expertise are improving, and so are the morbidity statistics.

More and more medical clinics are including this procedure as viable therapy.

Medicare now approves cryosurgery for use in prostate cancer treatment. Many health plans also are realizing the effectiveness of this technique and are approving its use.

Chapter 15

My Path

I am somewhat reluctant to describe my situation and the treatment solution I chose. Since each man must make his own analysis according to his own unique situation and identify his personal biases toward the problem he confronts, I do not wish to influence anyone. During my own initial readings I was aware that a persuasive book had a strong effect on my feelings and thinking. This is the stressful time when one will be most receptive to what one reads and learns. I want to warn the reader against this as he reads of my experience. I worry that a reader may decide that what I decided is what he needs, when that might prove to be inappropriate for his actual condition.

Nevertheless, in order to incorporate all these ideas, treatments and Treatment Option Charts into some semblance of order, I will share my own journey with you. You will see how I reviewed my original messy option decision charts, tables, and future treatment option considerations to arrive at a treatment that was comfortable for me, my outlook and psychology, yet was valid for the clinical conditions I was facing.

I have mentioned before that the final choice comes down to each individual's personal fears, desires and emotional responses to all the basic issues and physical conditions he faces. Constructing the charts helped me to sort things out and reduce confusion. After I did this, I was then able to focus on what treatments my particular condition actually allowed. By following my path and the rationale behind my ultimate choice, you may be able to find your way through the maze to a treatment choice that is appropriate and satisfying for you.

In preparing my Treatment Option Charts I educated myself in ways that I would not have done if I had merely followed directions from a couple of physicians. What the exercise did for me was to clarify in my mind *all* the treatment options open to me, the success statistics of the potential treatments, the side effects each option had, and what I should expect in the future.

I hope that if you spend time considering all the paths and options available for you, you will arrive at the understanding which provides the confidence that will add immeasurably to the success of your treatment choice.

I am a strong believer in the idea that a fully informed and confident patient will have superior treatment results.

I realize that, in the long run, any treatment that does the job is a good treatment. But one's future may be decided by what does *not* work for you. Of course, how does one know what works and what doesn't until the therapies are applied? It is like Will Rogers' comment about stock market investing: He advised people to buy only stocks that double in price, then sell them,... and if they don't double in price, don't buy them in the first place! For us, the task is to choose the treatment that truly works "in the first place" and to avoid all the others.

I was 61 when my tumor was discovered. I was otherwise very healthy and soon to be married. My physicians believed my clinical stage was a T1c or at worst a T2a. My Gleason type was a 3, with the second most common tumor cell also a 3. Thus, my Gleason score was a 6, a fairly common value. The tumor was on the small side, meaning its volume was far less than 5 percent of the prostate volume, hence the low stage value. It was located in the apex of my prostate, so I did not fear any surgical complications that might be of concern if it were located near the bladder. But tumor material located in the prostate apex tends to escape more often than from other locations.

From these basic numbers you can see that my treatment options lie in Figure 7.

But, I did have a PSA value of 10 and a 20 percent ploidy number, meaning that watchful waiting was not an option for me, as the tumor could be more aggressive than one might wish. Orchiectomy and alternative therapies were obviously not appropriate for my age, health, and tumor condition. Thus, I removed treatment options 1, 2, and 7 from consideration.

On Figure 7 you can see that for a 60-year-old in the green band of exceptional health for a T2 stage, the primary treatment options open are surgery, external beam X-ray radiation, proton beam radiation, brachytherapy, and cryosurgery. These options are indicated by the white circles. Note that there are no secondary treatment white diamonds on my color path. These are not needed unless a patient is staged T3 or T4. I did have, as adjuvant/co-partner, the white squares indicating combined hormone therapy as a preparation therapy for whatever primary treatment I decided upon.

Now, I admit that I have an aversion to the idea of surgery. I do not know why this is so. I studied the Partin nomogram shown as Figure 10. I saw that for a person with a PSA of 10, Gleason score 6, staged even as optimistically as T2a, I had only a 62 percent chance that the tumor would (pathologically) be shown to be confined within my prostate, despite what my physicians might (clinically) estimate my stage to be. This meant that there was a 38 percent chance that it had escaped from the prostate already! I have highlighted the relevant numbers for my case in Figure 10. You will remember that I wrote earlier that most tumors are clinically understaged, and upon removal are shown to be higher in stage than was originally estimated. This factor weighed heavily on my thoughts for some time.

To dispel them, I obtained a multispectral MRI of my prostate and pelvis. I wanted to see if tumor material was actually on or outside the prostate capsule wall. This new and very accurate MRI technique did reveal the possibility of "extension," meaning there were some clues that the tumor material was creeping along the wall of the prostate, and thus we were no longer confident that my tumor was completely confined. We were not 100 percent sure that this was the case, but if it turned out that tumor material had already escaped, then perhaps I was really a stage higher than a T2a, perhaps a T3a! In such a case the Partin nomogram offered even lower statistics for success with surgery. The MRI, however, proved that there was no tumor involvement in my seminal vesicles or lymph nodes, a comforting and reassuring discovery.

These factors caused me to lean away from a surgical prostatectomy operation.

Yet, I had to consider the aspects of compromising my choice of future treatments by my choice of primary treatments (see Figure 9). With surgery, I knew that if the tumor were truly confined within the prostate I had an excellent chance of total success. If a recurrence were to occur several years down the line, I would still have *all* the secondary treatment options open to me. In my visits to clinics and during my treatment, I was to meet many, many men who were undergoing radiation treatments for cancer that had returned or had not been fully excised by surgery.

With the choice of radiation as my primary treatment I knew my future options would be compromised, because future radiation treatments would be severely limited or ruled out altogether, and "salvage" surgery would be more difficult, with increased side effects.

The side effects of impotence and incontinence from surgery disturbed me also, but I rationalized that these statistics were compiled in part from many men who were older and weaker than I, perhaps no longer potent anyway, and most likely not newly married! (I have since learned that this was, in part, an erroneous conclusion. The morbidity statistics result from the treatment more or less regardless of patient age.)

The morbidity considerations weighed on me when I considered cryosurgery. It appears that the short term result of freezing yields more than 70 percent impotence, with perhaps only half of such patients regaining potency after a year or so. Some 10 percent of such patients have incontinence problems with this therapy. I was too young and active to take this statistic in stride. There are also a number of other side effects connected with this technique, as outlined in Chapter 14.

Should I keep cryosurgery as a back-up treatment in the event of a failed surgery or radiation? If I did, the side effects of cryosurgery as a "salvage treatment" were even worse. Indeed, incontinence approaches 50 percent when cryosurgery is used as a secondary treatment.

These considerations forced me to consider radiation of some kind as my primary treatment, treatment options 4a, 4b, or 5 on Figure 9. Now, I have an aversion to radiation, too. I do not like the idea of high-energy particles whizzing through my body. Was I really willing to risk serious radiation damage to normal tissue in my pelvis? But I knew it would be wisest and safest to treat me conservatively as a T2b stage, as indicated by the MRI, and not as a lesser stage patient. Radiation would be effective and appropriate for a T2b stage patient.

Compared to surgery, the radiation treatment options seemed to me to offer lesser likelihood of incontinence and impotence, and to have less potential for recurrence. I reviewed the survival statistics for the radiation possibilities.

Traditional, old-fashioned, external beam X-ray treatments did not excite me. Ten-year survival curves were not as good as I had originally been led to believe. There was a reasonable chance that I would be dead in a decade. To be dead at age 72? In this era? I have too much to do before I leave the stage! I eliminated traditional X-ray radiation from consideration. This left me with 3D conformal external beam radiation, proton beam radiation, or brachytherapy as treatment options.

I concentrated on these three possibilities and looked

into all the statistics associated with them. The MRI indicated the wisdom of treating me as at least a T2b, even though I knew the tumor was small enough to be clinically staged as a T2a, if not a T1c. But the possibility of an extension worried me.

I learned that 3D conformal beam radiation would cover the area of possible extension, while still targeting the main tumor bulk shown by the sonogram, MRI, and CAT scan imaging. I knew, also, that the radiation would attack any unseen micro-tumor sites lying within the prostate. In conformal beam radiation a computer model of the prostate is tailor-made specifically to each man's gland. The radiation doses are directed to give the maximum dose to the tumor site, with lower doses out to the edges of the prostate. In my case, a "halo" of about one centimeter beyond the wall of the prostate would be radiated. This would kill any tumor material that might be creeping along the prostate capsule wall. But it would also endanger some of the critical nerves that are near the prostate.

I then looked into brachytherapy as my primary treatment. Seed implantation has become so accurate that it competes with surgery and external beam radiation. Seed implantation alone would offer an effective alternative to surgery so long as all tumor material was still located within the prostate. But the possibility of an extension of tumor growth argued against using brachytherapy alone for my primary treatment.

I was now forced to consider the combination of 3D conformal external beam radiation *combined* with seed implantation as my primary treatment. I learned that the combination of the two radiation treatments had the potential to be as effective as surgery, and, in my case, to be more thorough than seed implantation alone. I also realized that new alternative therapies might be available in a few years. That is, if I were to have a failure, with a rising PSA, I felt that I would soon have hormones, potential anti-angiogenesis treatments, chemotherapy, vaccinations or genetic solutions for prostate cancer to fall back on. If I were to choose this approach, I reasoned that I had, at the very least, purchased myself half a decade of time for the new alternative therapies to be made available. Lastly, I still had surgery or cryosurgery as salvage surgeries in case of a failure, despite the unhappy side effects. I would also be eligible for some very limited additional seed implantation if residual tumor material remained in my prostate.

My thoughts were now seriously directed toward 3D conformal external beam radiation *combined* with seed implantation, to be implemented by doctors Mack Roach III, Katsuto Shinohara and Eric Vigneault at the University of California Medical Center at San Francisco. I was impressed by their thoroughness, precision and patient attention.

All during the time period of my study and repeated visits to various physicians I was on triple hormone anti-androgen therapy, a treatment indicated by the white squares on the option chart. In fact, I remained on this therapy for ten months, longer than many physicians think is wise. But I wished to damage and shrink the tumor as much as possible. I wanted to reduce the volume of my prostate so that a surgeon or radiologist would have the smallest gland possible to deal with. I also wanted to make the tumor less resistant to radiation, if my ultimate decision favored a radiation treatment. The hormone treatment was so effective that when I appeared for my primary treatment, my PSA had dropped from 10ng/ml to 0.02ng/ml! If you are contemplating hormone treatment, discuss it with your physicians. Some radiologists do not favor hormonal use as pre-treatment for seed implantation. (See Chapter 17.)

During the period of my investigations, more long-term data came out to support the concept that conformal beam EBRT combined with seed treatment would offer powerful competition to surgery. In fact, the data presented in the 1997 monograph by Stamey (see bibliography) show the *combined* radiation treatment to be by far the most successful radiation treatment available to any patient who is staged as T1 or T2. And brachytherapy now has eight-year statistical data which compare favorably with surgical prostatectomy data.

I also looked into proton beam radiation at Loma Linda University Medical Center in Southern California. I was so impressed with this concept that I made several visits to the center, talking with the physicians in charge of this therapy. I was pleased with the attention I received from Dr. Carl Rossi, Jr. I liked the way the killing power of the proton beam was delivered solely to the prostate and the way it minimized damage to tissue anywhere else. This therapy is also provided in combination with 3D conformal beam radiation.

I could receive 25 days of conformal beam radiation at either facility, combined with seeds or with proton beam radiation. Since the strength of EBRT in either treatment would be identical, it was a matter of seeds vs. proton beams. I was almost equally keen on each program. In favor of the combined proton beam therapy was the fact that no permanently implanted metal seeds were involved. Seeds, in the event of future salvage surgery, would make it far more difficult for a surgeon to remove my prostate. In discussions with physicians at both centers, I was told that the competing treatments would most likely offer identical results regarding morbidity and success. I was down to flipping coins. That is how far I had come from my original treatment dilemma! At last, I had worked my way through the maze and narrowed my choices to two.

After considerable thought, I decided on the 3D conformal external beam radiation combined with seed implantation. There are several centers across the nation that specialize in these treatments (see Appendix F.) After visiting more than half a dozen medical centers during the year, I became more and more impressed with the University of

California San Francisco Medical Center. I liked the physicians there, who, while being on the cutting edge of a new technology, were still patient and attentive to my incessant inquiries.

In early 1998, I received 25 daily 3D conformal external beam X-ray treatments at UCSF Medical Center, followed immediately by the implantation of 91 radioactive iodine seeds. The search for my treatment was finished. In fact, my treatment was finished.

The reader can apply the same kind of analysis to his own condition. Start with *your* basic statistics and health situation. *Put aside all thoughts of the treatment options that others may face.* Eliminate the obviously inappropriate treatment options. Now you have narrowed down the possibilities to only a few. Consider the side effects, the morbidity statistics of these treatments, the limitations regarding future treatment options, your personal preferences, fears, likes and dislikes.

Does your treatment path make sense to you? Does it make sense to your physicians? Are you emotionally comfortable with it? What about the future for you? Are your physicians encouraging to you in this regard?

Make your final choice when you are confident and comfortable. This will go a long way toward assuring you of success in ridding your body of cancer. The next chapter will show you paths that other patients might follow.

Remember This

In this chapter I attempted to put myself in your shoes. I tried to show you how I overcame my emotions and anxieties by developing my decision charts.

My path, the development of my Treatment Option Charts, the consideration of all the tradeoffs involved, led me to the decision rationale for my treatment. This process

gave me confidence that I would be successfully treated.

Take the time to review Chapters 7, 8 and 9 again and apply that information to what I have written in this chapter. I think you will find that the clouds will be clearing and that you will determine a rationale for treatment as I did.

Chapter 16

Other Paths

In the previous chapter I outlined the conditions I faced, my concerns and desires and the rationale that led up to what I felt was a valid path for me to follow. I must stress that this choice may not be the same for a man with different basic conditions, who is in a different age group, or who has a different level of health.

Let me outline a possible path for a man who has a basic condition similar to mine, but who is much younger than I was when cancer was detected. This exercise may help explain how to use the Treatment Option Charts to arrive at a different treatment procedure.

Let us say that a man has a Gleason score of 6, is clinically staged as a T2a, has a PSA of 5 ng/ml, is 45 years old and very healthy in all other respects.

This patient can consider surgery, external beam radiation, seed implantation, and cryosurgery, as shown by the primary treatment white circles in Figure 7. He is too young and healthy to even consider the watchful waiting treatment option, and his tumor is so contained that even if he is understaged he should not consider the alternative therapies.

He may feel that life has played a trick on him. Because so many new therapies are coming soon, he may feel that he will be the last man to have a prostatectomy. This is a very unnerving thought. Yet, he is young and has the potential for a long life ahead of him. He probably has family responsibilities to consider. What should he do?

If he opts for surgery he will have several significant concerns. The incidence of death because of the surgical procedures is negligible. If he has a good surgeon all tumor cells should be successfully removed. Thus, he may concentrate on the chances for impotence (which for a 45-year-old may be of great concern), and of incontinence (which is most likely a minor possibility). He should be fully aware of the real morbidity statistics, as discussed in Chapter 8.

If he is healthy and chooses surgery, he has one great advantage over any other option before him: The other treatment options are all still available to him if he does have a recurrence of cancer, discovered over the years during his post-operative PSA testing. He will have external beam radiation open to him as well as cryosurgery and seed implantation. These future options are shown in Figure 9.

Now, let us consider the choices open to him if he chooses seed implantation or the combination of external beam radiation with brachytherapy as his primary treatment. Maybe, like me, he is sobered by the morbidity considerations and not too keen on any surgical procedure. Even with nerve-sparing surgical techniques at the major specialty clinics, he still faces the potential of impotence. But in the case of a 45-year-old man who has some 30 to 40 years of life left, brachytherapy may not be the best option. Can we be sure that seed implantation will do the trick over such a long time? We do not have records that can prove this. For a man over 60 years of age, such as myself, this seems a very reasonable choice, as it is likely that he will be suffering other major health issues within a decade anyway, so a failure here may not loom so large.

For a 45-year-old who has a failure ten years after radiation, what is he to use as backup treatment? He has most likely used up his radiation allotment so a full secondary radiation treatment is not open to him. He has closed that future treatment option, for the most part.

Salvage surgery will be open to him, but surgery after radiation is more difficult than it is as the primary therapy. Cryosurgery will be open to him, but this, too, has more unfavorable side effects than when it is the primary therapy.

So, the dilemma this man faces is how to fulfill his longevity cancer-free, or, in the case of a failure, not to compromise future treatment options. If he chooses radiation or seed implantation, he may hope that, in the event of a recurrence, the new DNA or anti-angiogenesis drugs will appear within a decade to solve the problem. If they are not available, he will face increased downside morbidity as a result of any secondary treatment he may require.

If he chooses surgery in the first place, he runs the risks of incontinence and impotence morbidities as a result. But if his surgery is done at a major clinic, is clean and accurate, he will be free of cancer and will probably suffer only minor downside morbidity effects.

For the 45-year-old, surgery could be a valid primary treatment choice as shown by the Treatment Option Charts and the Future Treatment Option Chart. His decision is now governed only by his attitude toward surgery and related morbidity statistics.

Finally, let's examine the situation for a man who is in poor or frail health and is over 70 years of age. Suppose, also, that his Gleason score is an 8. His PSA is 20 ng/ml. His staging is a T3. This man is in trouble, well on his way to having a metastasizing tumor to deal with. What options are open to him? This man's solutions appear in Figure 8.

Most likely he is no longer sexually active, so his concerns about potency are much reduced over those of the younger man. His health may not allow a surgery, and even if it would allow such a stress to his system, the staging and PSA value tells us that surgery may be insufficient to rid him of cancer. Even brachytherapy may be questionable, as it is most useful for localized tumors, less so for those that have escaped from the prostate.

The white circles on the Treatment Option Chart show that his main treatment choices are external beam radiation, orchiectomy, and/or alternative therapies, or some combination of these treatments. Most likely, hormone therapies also will be used, as indicated by the white squares. External beam radiation will cover the entire prostate as well as the area surrounding it, where escaped cancer cells are most likely to reside. Furthermore, if tumor material has migrated to other organs or to his bones, new diagnostic tests such as Prostascint scans and MRI imaging may identify their locations. Here, external beam radiation can help. Hormone treatments and new clinical trial drugs would also be an important factor in his treatment.

Treatment Option Decision Charts, coupled with the Future Treatment Option Chart, will guide him toward the reasonable options open to him. At the very least, they will steer him away from treatments that are inappropriate.

After you study the charts you need to confront your emotions regarding any of the treatments. Each man is different in his fears, his priorities and desires. In the long run, the choice of treatment is up to the individual. I hope that my Treatment Option Charts help sort out what is important for *your* case so that you can reach a comfortable and confident decision based on reason and what is appropriate for you. The rest is up to you.

Remember This

A careful study of the Treatment Option Charts will help guide your decision. The right course for one man may be wrong for another. This is the critical concept in this decision guide. Each man must make his own treatment decision. No one can make it for him. To be assured that an appropriate treatment option is chosen, he must know all the factors involved in that decision.

Chapter 17

What About Hormone Treatments?

You will wake up at night, sweating and kicking off the bedcovers. You then retreat to the warmth as you begin to shiver. The hot flashes also happen throughout the day. It may be embarrassing. You may get cranky, too. I did not get cranky, or so I would like to think. Perhaps those around me were polite and kept the knowledge from me that I was cantankerous. Your libido will disappear within a few months, and you will have little interest in sex. But you will understand and appreciate what many of our wives and women friends go through in the course of menopause. You are sharing many of their symptoms.

Why would any man subject himself to this? There are valid reasons to do this.

In 1966, Dr. Charles Huggins won a well-deserved Nobel Prize for his earlier discovery and proof that in order to grow, prostate cancer requires male hormones called androgens. The hormone testosterone is the main one implicated in prostate cancer growth. Cut off that supply and the cancer will stop growing, at least temporarily. Physicians do this by prescribing hormones and medications that cause a "combined hormonal blockage" (CHB) of the body's testosterone production. Some are injected and some are taken orally. These are often combined.

Until recently the use of hormones as treatment was reserved for patients whose cancer had spread to other tissues within the body. Or perhaps tumor cells were not fully removed by radiation or surgery, and hormonal treatments were employed as a secondary line of treatment. All of this is now changing, as more evidence appears suggesting that hormone use as a pre-treatment has significant advantages for the ultimate outcome, whether the patient is treated by surgery or radiation.

Some physicians do not advocate use of hormone treatments, but many physicians now like the patient to undergo perhaps six to ten months of hormone blockage, which is called "anti-androgen therapy," or "complete androgen blockage." The term "anti-androgen" therapy is often used in the literature to describe the hormones which counteract cancer-stimulating hormones such as testosterone.

When this anti-androgen therapy is used prior to upcoming surgery or radiation, it is called "neoadjuvant hormonal therapy," meaning it precedes and combines with surgical or radiation intervention. (The term "adjuvant" hormonal intervention signifies use as a secondary therapy during and after a primary treatment). In my case I was on three medications for ten months, at which time my tumor had "downsized" to the extent that it could no longer be seen clearly on the standard sonogram.

The shrinkage of my tumor would make a surgeon's job easier. Indeed, a number of on-going studies show that among patients who receive three or more months of combined hormonal therapy (CHT) prior to a radical prostatectomy, about one-third more have negative surgical margins (no evidence of cancer growth near the wall of the prostate), than patients who have surgery with *no* prior hormone therapy. This means that any cancer cells that *may* have resided on the margins of the prostate wall were removed because of the hormone treatments.

Hormone therapy reduces the radiologist's target size (and also hopefully removes any micrometastatic cancer deposits) and at the same time "softens up" the tumor tissue so that radiation becomes more effective in killing it. Evidence is mounting that hormone treatments prior to radiation provide an improvement in progression-free survival time (meaning no evidence of a recurrence) and often in over-all survival time.

If you have an exceptionally large prostate, your physician may require hormone therapy just to reduce your prostate size so that he can safely radiate it without undue exposure to other parts of your body. If your prostate shrinks by 50 percent, the radiation dosage density to that area doubles, as does its killing power.

Of all hormone-sensitive cancers, prostate cancer is the most sensitive to hormonal manipulation and control; a positive response to combined therapy is noted in more than 85 percent of men. For some patients, hormone therapy is so successful that, after treatment, no cancer can be found in the prostate after removal of the gland by surgery. In fact, this success rate may be as high as 1 in 4. Nevertheless, most physicians believe that hormone therapy alone does not actually remove cancer from your system, but instead merely reduces the tumor to an indistinguishable volume. PSA monitoring during and after hormone treatment will be the first tip-off if hormone therapy is failing to control tumor growth.

Although most physicians regard hormone therapy as non-curative, some urologists do recommend triple hormone blockage as a *primary* treatment for localized tumor conditions because of the evidence that cancer cells are actually killed, not just put into remission of some kind. Advocates believe that the *combined* effect of triple hormone blockage sets into action a process called "apoptosis," meaning cell death. This subject is very controversial, contains risks, and merits discussion with your physician. But increasingly, over the past two years, physicians are recognizing that triple hormonal blockage can be a valuable preconditioning treatment for radiation and surgery. The drugs used in this triple hormone approach are now:

Lupron, or Zoladex or Goserelin (injected drugs): These drugs are called luteinizing hormone-releasing hormone agonists (LHRH), and they suppress testicular androgen.

Casodex, or Eulexin (taken orally): These prescriptions are anti-androgens that the body tolerates well.

> **Proscar,** or Finasteride (taken orally): These chemicals block enzymes that produce testosterone. This prescription will have little impact on sexual activity, while the other two medicines will lower your desire and abilities.

Many physicians use what is called "intermittent hormonal therapy." The patient is given triple hormone blockage for, say a year to eighteen months, then taken off the hormones until his PSA values rise above what is regarded as normal for his age. Then he is again placed on the hormone treatment. Such patients live a much more satisfactory life than those who remain continuously on the hormones. There are cases of men living a normal life for a decade or more with this on-and-off therapy.

If you are unlucky, and your cancer was discovered only after it had spread to other sites in your body, it will be mandatory that you treat the condition with hormones to at least stabilize growth, if not stop it entirely in a few cases. With some patients, the CHB technique is so powerful that, after six to nine months, a clinical stage T3 cancer is downstaged to a pathological stage T2, thus opening up the possibilities for treatment as the lower staged condition. Some men in advanced states of metastasis require an orchiectomy (removal of one's testes) in order to stop the production of testosterone altogether. While this may seem drastic, one needs to give thoughtful and balanced consideration to such a step, especially since we are talking about life and death.

Short of an orchiectomy, men with advanced cancer can control its spread (and retard further spreading to a certain extent) with hormones that block the effects of testosterone. Sad to say, however, at this time, hormone treatment is not completely effective over extended periods of time. But curiously, in some 5 percent to 10 percent of patients with advanced cancer, CHT has been shown not only to reduce cancer symptoms but actually to eliminate cancer from their prostates. The normal pattern, however, is that in a few years the tumor finds ways to grow without the need for testosterone. The tumor material, no matter where it lies in your body, is now "refractory," meaning it is resistant to the hormone effects and no longer responds to hormonal control. This fact bolsters evidence that the earlier the hormonal therapy begins, the longer it takes for hormonal resistance to develop. At present there are few truly effective treatments for men with metastatic, hormonally insensitive cancer, and chemotherapy will be required. Chemotherapy does extend life and palliates (meaning to relieve) your condition.

For the majority of men who are staged as T1's or T2's, the use of hormone treatments as assisting therapy does three good things:

1. It buys you some time to work out the primary treatment that is most comfortable for you. You can safely remain on hormone treatments for many months, if not a year or so, so long as regular blood tests indicate your body is tolerating this therapy properly.

2. This treatment reduces the size of the prostate and the tumor. This helps your surgeon or radiologist. Normally, the prostate will shrink by 50 percent within a few months. This is advantageous because radiologists and many surgeons prefer a smaller target. It makes surgery a far less difficult procedure. According to many physicians, if you have an abnormally large prostate, you *must* use hormones to shrink it.

3. It markedly improves your survival statistics if your primary treatment is radiation. While your prostate is shrinking, the tumor itself seems to "downsize," and even "downstage" its condition, making it more susceptible to radiation. It appears that tumor tissue, becomes less and less resistant to radiation, compared to normal tissue. More and more evidence is appearing that the *combined* use of anti-androgen therapy before, during, and after radiation

treatment has a synergistic effect that dramatically increases survivability and helps completely eradicate cancer.

Many believe a new standard of treatment for men with higher risk disease soon will be therapy combining hormonal suppression drugs with radiation. Studies show that fewer than half the men with PSA's greater than 10 ng/ml, Gleason scores greater than 7, and clinical staging greater than T2b are disease free after five years when they received radiation alone. Such a patient may not be a good candidate for surgery, but if hormonal suppression is combined with radiation, the disease-free statistic is impressive. After three years, in one study, rising PSA levels were detected in 81 percent of patients treated with radiation alone, versus only 15 percent of patients given hormone therapy with radiation.

It is obvious why more and more physicians are using hormone therapy for pre-treatment of cancer, often requesting it for up to six months prior to surgery or radiation. It makes sense to "break down" and downsize your tumor, especially if you choose radiation of some kind to eliminate it. An even field of radiation to your prostate, for instance, will be far more efficient in killing dispersed cancer (dispersed perhaps into microscopic foci) than it might be in eliminating a solid tumor of some volume. The day is coming when neoadjuvant hormone therapy may become standard practice to prepare the patient for his primary therapy. More and more evidence is appearing that hormone therapy is most effective when it is started early, when the number of cancer cells is at the lowest point.

At the present time, however, there are some relevant arguments against the use of hormone therapy. Some surgeons believe that pre-treatment with combined hormone therapy makes it more difficult for them to clearly identify the prostate boundary during the surgery, that the margins become indistinct or "fuzzy." A number of brachytherapists are concerned that if the prostate is shrunk too much before the implantation of the seeds, the seeds are compacted too closely and could injure the urethra, or possibly the rectum. External beam radiation on a very small prostate could also over-radiate the rectum. These radiologists consider hormone use only *after* implantation and radiation.

There are a number of health side effects in hormonal therapy which you need to discuss with your physician. The side effects for which your physician will be watching include general weakness, disruption of liver function, muscle deterioration, alterations in bone density, and possibly heart difficulties. He will monitor the side effects of hormone therapy by ordering a full blood test every other month. Obtain baseline liver and blood tests prior to beginning hormonal therapy. I wish I had done this, as I do not know what my testosterone level was prior to hormone use, even though my testosterone level is now in the "normal" range.

Remember This

The medical industry is gathering more and more case history evidence which shows the advantages of pre-treatment with combined hormonal therapy. Within a few more years, no doubt, even the skeptics in the profession will advocate this use. Many believe that soon it will become standard practice with any and all treatment options.

Combining hormonal blockage drugs with surgery or radiation reduces the risk of metastatic cancer, and increases survival. Improved results from these techniques may require up to three years of hormone therapy. It appears that hormone therapy is most successful on tumors that are below a certain size and less effective for larger tumors.

Prolonged use of combined hormonal blockage medi-

cines can result in a chemical impotence. This can also disrupt aspects of basic body chemistry. CHT use must be monitored for this eventuality with frequent blood tests.

Many men believe that all men treated with this therapy will eventually develop a refractory tumor condition where the hormones no longer have a controlling effect on tumor growth. This is not true. Hormone resistance is not inevitable in every man, especially if the tumor size is small to begin with. Many men have hormonal success lasting up to two decades.

Ask your physician if this treatment is right for you. At the very least, a few months on it will buy you some time so you can study all the aspects of the potential treatments that are open to you

Chapter 18

What About Diet?

Americans are among the fattest people on earth. How we got this way is best left to historians, as our dietary evolution is very complicated and is interwoven with the flow of our history. We are now at a pinnacle of obesity, and our health statistics show this every year. In the 50- to 70-year age group for men, we are twice as likely to be obese as people in their 20's. It is likely that this fact is related to the statistics for prostate cancer. The Center for Disease Control and Prevention indicates that excess weight kills more than a quarter of a million Americans prematurely every year, by contributing to heart attacks, strokes, high blood pressure, diabetes, and possibly many cancers. Scientists now believe that at least one third of all cancers are related in some way to what we eat and drink.

It is more than mere coincidence, it seems to me, that American men have one of the highest prostate cancer rates in the world, while Japanese men have rates among the lowest. But when Japanese men move to the U.S. and adopt the traditional American diet, their prostate cancer rates rise to match the national average. The scientific community is only now beginning to pay serious attention to the role that diet plays in preventing or fighting cancer.

There are things we all need to know about diet. Not just we patients, but our physicians and dieticians also need to know far more about the proper use of diet to generate and maintain good health. The field is not exact at the present time. We are learning about foods and drinks to avoid; new information about carcinogenic substances in common foods and beverages is revealed almost daily.

Dr. William Fair, a prostate cancer specialist engaged in diet studies at Sloan-Kettering Cancer Center in New York, believes that prostate cancer may be a nutritional disease. He observes that the occurrence of incipient microfocal cancer is about the same worldwide, but that tumors arise mostly in the more developed countries that have diets rich in fat. Former Surgeon General C. Everett Koop believes that some 70 percent of Americans are dying from diseases related to our diet.

So, if diet influences the initiation and growth of cancer, then it is obvious that it has its most powerful effect on men in socicties where a particular diet is a permanent life style. In our culture, once a tumor has begun, we should not expect to control cancer by diet alone. But Fair has evidence that patients who follow his diet regimens show at least an *inhibition* of cancer growth, and he believes that the patient who follows such a regimen is empowered by his taking an active role in his own medical outcome, because this is psychologically important to help control or defeat cancer. Spend some time studying this subject if it interests you, as it should, and talk with your physicians about it.

You will read all sorts of things about diet, even that *all* diseases can be controlled by diet, vitamins, exercise, proper sleep, etc., but little is really known or understood on a scientific basis. There are, however, a number of substantiated dietary facts that might impact prostate cancer growth and can be stated with some certainty:

Diets with high fat intake increase the chances of cancer growth.
Fruits and vegetables help reduce cancer growth.
Diets high in fiber and soy products yield reduced cancer statistics.
Green tea has been found to be a cancer retardant.

You want to eat foods that stimulate your immune system, and avoid foods or drinks that depress it. In our lives we take our immune system almost for granted, like breathing. We give little thought to whether or not it is functioning correctly. Obviously it is functioning correctly, and this is made clear when we recover from a cold, the flu, or a more serious infection. But think about this for a moment: *Our immune system can fail us only once,* so we should do everything we can to maximize its efficiency, especially if we have cancer.

Fiber:

There is no proper scientific study that has produced truly scientific evidence that diets high in fruits and fiber result in lower prostate cancer statistics. But researchers believe that fiber promotes clearance of fats and waste products from the body more rapidly, thus reducing opportunities for cancer to begin. This is why many physicians recommend eating a breakfast of cereal, such as All-Bran, bran flakes, raisin bran, or oatmeal. This easy habit will provide most of your fiber requirements, from 10 to 20 grams per day. If you also eat several pieces of fruit during the day, you should get all the fiber you need.

We know that foods high in fiber, such as fruits, whole grains, and oatmeal do play an important role in reducing colon cancer. There is evidence to suggest that fiber has an effect upon the growth of other cancers as well. Fiber in the digestive tract improves elimination of waste products. Many believe that efficient elimination of body wastes minimizes the chemicals that may cause DNA damages. Damaged DNA is required for cancer to begin.

Vegetables:

A recent study indicates that men who have diets heavy in tomato products, such as cooked tomatoes, tomato sauce, pizza, etc., have reduced cancer incidence. Lycopene is the phytochemical that gives tomatoes their red color, and it appears that it gives a degree of cancer protection. A large randomized study by Harvard University reveals that men with diets rich in lycopene were least likely to develop prostate cancer. It concludes that not only is it possible that lycopene may prevent prostate cancer, but it may also be useful in *treating* the condition. Curiously, it is the most abundant carotenoid in the prostate. As yet there is no clinical proof that, once a tumor has been discovered, a change in diet will remove the cancer. It may be that certain foods prevent microscopic cancers from developing in the first place, but once a real tumor has begun, the benefits from diet are diminished.

Other vegetables that contain significant amounts of phytochemicals are cabbage, celery, red peppers, kale, lemons, onions, and strawberries.

High Fat Diet:

A recent study at Harvard University indicates that men who consumed a diet high in animal fats had a 79 percent increased risk of advanced cancer, as compared to men with the lowest intake of such fats. Fat intake seems to determine whether or not prostate tumors remain small and non-threatening, or progress into life-threatening conditions. High fat levels in your body after you have been diagnosed with or treated for cancer may be dangerous. Fat seems to stimulate tumor cells to evade the immune system. High consumption of fat is already well verified as promoting breast cancer and colon cancer. Recent studies indicate that the effect of fat in promotion of prostate cancer is even stronger. Consumption of polyunsaturated fats commonly found in the American diet probably fuels the growth and spread of prostate cancer in men.

High saturated fat intake during one's lifetime has been statistically linked to prostate cancer. It may be that most men have incipient or latent cancer sites, and this incidence is the same for American men and Japanese men. Autopsy studies of men from different cultures suggest this is the case. In countries such as Japan, where traditional diets are low in fat and high in fiber, statistics for *developed* tumors are low. Japanese men, when they do develop tumors, tend to have less aggressive forms of cancer than do American men.

As Asian countries become "westernized" with a dietary increase of red meat and fat, the statistics of prostate cancer rise along with the increase in meat consumption.

This makes sense. If red meat raises the production of testosterone in men, and prostate cancer requires testosterone to grow, then it follows that a society that consumes red meat as a normal part of its diet will be faced with higher prostate cancer statistics than societies that seldom eat red meat. In Sloan-Kettering laboratories, mice with transplanted human tumors were divided into two groups. One ate a diet high in fats, and the other ate a low fat diet. The group that consumed the highest amount of fat had the faster tumor growth rates.

You must not eliminate all fats from your diet, as there are a number of *essential fatty acids* that are required for proper vitamin absorption. This issue must be discussed with your physician before you become a full vegetarian or vegan. No doubt your doctor will agree that lowering your intake of red meat, eggs, and dairy products is a wise move. At the very least, the reduction may encourage you to eat more vegetables to fill the void. The Harvard School of Public Health conducted studies that suggest that red meat, dairy fat, egg yolks, and creamy salad dressings are significant dietary concerns for cancer. The National Cancer Institute has recommendations for diets that may resist cancer growth.

Soy Products:

Regarding the use of soy products such as tofu, tempeh, soybeans, soymilk, and miso, there is anecdotal as well as clinical evidence to consider. Soy products contain the phytochemical genistein, an isoflavone that is shown to combat a number of cancers. In many Asian societies, red meat is a rarity, while consumption of green tea and soy products is common in everyday life. In Japan, with twice the number of smokers as in the U.S., the lung cancer rate is only one-half of ours. Japan has a breast cancer rate only one-sixth of ours and a prostate cancer rate of one-*thirtieth* of ours! We know that soybean products provide healthy protein. Soy foods may lower blood cholesterol, therefore reducing heart disease. Soy-related plants most likely provide a measure of protection against cancers of all kinds.

It appears that genistein blocks one of the major mechanisms by which cancer cells become hormone refractory. (A refractory tumor is one that no longer responds to hormone control). Perhaps this substance offers a measure of protection against the building of new blood vessels to a tumor. In laboratory experiments, high doses of genistein have been shown to kill cancer cells. Isoflavones are plant estrogens called phytoestrogens, and in clinical tests it appears that these estrogens have an effect upon hormone-related cancers, such as breast and prostate cancer. The most-used breast cancer treatment is tamoxifen, and it works in ways similar to the isoflavones.

Soybeans and soybean products are not traditional in American diets, as they are in Asian countries. We now are advised by many clinicians to eat one cup of soybean product daily. Soy products replace the protein that our bodies miss when we reduce consumption of red meat. Soy products can easily be added to fruit drinks and to recipes. The Iowa Soybean Promotion Board offers a free cookbook with dozens of recipes. (Iowa Soybean Promotion Board, 4554 N.W. 114th Street, Urbandale, IA, 50322-5410).

While large-scale randomized trials are required to prove the anti-cancer effects of soy products, a 1989 study published in *Cancer Research* reviewed 8,000 Hawaiian men of Japanese ancestry. Those men who ate the most tofu had the lowest rates of prostate cancer. There is growing evidence that soy consumption arrests tumor growth, and if taken in high doses, may even kill prostate cancer cells. The UCLA/NCI Clinical Nutrition Research Unit in Los Angeles conducts clinical studies on diets high in soy protein for men with prostate cancer.

Green Tea:

Green tea appears to have anti-cancer qualities, and considerable research is being done on this substance. Green tea is high in catechins, powerful antioxidants. A University of Kansas study reveals that catechin anti-oxidants are 100 times more effective than vitamin C and 25 times more powerful than vitamin E. According to the *American Journal of Clinical Nutrition*, green tea also protects against heart disease. It is no substitute for a good cup of coffee, but we are advised to reduce coffee intake and to increase green tea consumption to more than three cups a day.

We read that a cancer patient must not eat fatty foods, red meat, drink coffee, use alcohol, or eat milk chocolate. Chocolate? Will the list of sacrifices we must endure never end? Well, it does seem to be unending. We should avoid fats, cut down on polyunsaturated oils, including canola, soybean, safflower, corn, cottonseed, and peanut oils. Olive oil, which is a monounsaturated fat, is the safest to use for cooking, and even this is a compromise. We need to watch carefully for fatty white meats of any kind, cheese, butter, egg yolks, mayonnaise, and all milk, yogurt, and sour cream containing fat. Substitute soy milk for your milk requirements. "Reduced fat" items are not enough. Buy only "fat-free" items to be sure you reduce fat consumption as much as possible.

I was 61 years old when my cancer was discovered. At the time, I was in good health and weighed ten pounds less than I did when I was in college. This can be explained, perhaps, by my loss of hair in the intervening years.

Nevertheless, for the past twenty years or so I have

maintained my weight to within plus or minus 5 pounds of 155 pounds. I am five feet ten inches tall. While I am not altogether pleased with how this weight is now distributed, I can take some pride in the fact that for the most part, I am pretty trim.

For the past two decades, I have exercised and watched my diet. Two decades ago I learned as much as I could about diet and its effect upon heart disease and health in general. I have maintained a kind of semi-Pritikin balance in my eating and drinking habits ever since.

While the studies by Pritikin, Cameron, Pauling and others show clearly that diet and good health are closely correlated, it seems that a diet structured to benefit the heart will also benefit the entire body in preventing or retarding cancer growth. Note that countries having a high incidence of heart disease also have a high incidence of prostate cancer.

Yet, I was diagnosed with cancer in 1997. After giving considerable attention to having a healthy heart, the enemy entered through the back door, so to speak, a situation that is a bit ironic. I have a friend who is a dedicated marathon runner, who ate a high fiber diet, yet still developed prostate cancer at age 57. Despite these contradictions, it makes sense to give attention to a proper diet and moderate eating and drinking habits if you have cancer of any kind, and even if you don't.

It is wise to discuss dietary matters with your oncologist, especially if you are overweight or out of shape. Clinical evidence indicates that the consumption of too much fatty food, refined sugar, salt, coffee and alcohol can encourage growth of cancer. Nutritionist Dr. Patrick Quillin believes that tumors are "sugar feeders."

The book by Kaltenbach, listed in the bibliography, has an informative chapter regarding diet and cancer. And the book by Dr. Anthony Sattilaro gives his own account of surviving advanced prostate cancer and the role he thinks diet played in his recovery.

The book by Morra and Potts, also listed in the bibliography, has information about dietary measures that are believed helpful for cancer patients. You must inform your physician about any decision you make to assist in treating your cancer with dietary measures. Many diet treatments in the past have been discredited by science and by succeeding years of study. Do not rely on diet alone, no matter how effective it may sound to you. Always consult your physicians in this regard.

Remember This

Some researchers refer to prostate cancer and heart disease as diseases of the affluent.

Heart patients and by-pass survivors are strongly advised to remove from their lives the factors that contributed to their condition: Stress, tobacco, and high-fat diets. We know these factors contribute to heart disease.

We also know there are dietary factors connected to cancer growth. The chapter on statistics and Figure 9, which indicates ten-year recurrence rates, suggest strongly that the chances of a recurrence are greater than those reported by the major clinics. If that is the case, isn't it wise to follow the advice given heart patients and do all you can to work toward a cancer-free future also?

Some clinicians believe that more than half of all prostate cancers could be prevented by changes in diet and lifestyle. By initiating new dietary habits you may find that you will live a lot longer, your heart with be stronger, and you may reduce risk of cancer of any kind.

Decrease the amount of dietary fat in your diet. Increase the levels of fruit and fiber you would normally consume. Increase your consumption of soy products. Reduce your

use of dairy products, such as whole milk, cheese, ice cream, and butter.

Every day your immune system protects your life. Your immune system can fail you only once. This being the case, is it not wise to assist your immune system in every way you can? It makes sense on many health fronts to eat more wisely as we become better informed on the subject.

What do you have to lose?

Chapter 19

What About Vitamins?

A good diet should provide enough vitamins for good health. The foods we eat and the vitamins we take are intended to maximize the efficiency of our immune system. Our immune system must confront and combat many types of foreign substances, such as bacteria, fungi, viruses, protozoa, and various parasites, as well as toxic substances that may enter our bodies. How can we expect to maintain good health without a proper immune system, hard at work, day and night? We should all maintain good dietary and vitamin habits from an early age, not delay these habits until illness strikes us.

Vitamins are profoundly important for proper metabolism and body functioning. The amounts of vitamins that are recommended are shown on all of our vitamin bottles. The "percent U.S. RDA" is the Federal Drug Administration's "recommended daily allowance" for a particular vitamin.

These are regarded as the *minimum* vitamin levels that we must maintain to insure proper health. Scientists know that vitamin deficiencies, even if very small, can seriously damage our systems. Many people believe that the RDA numbers are far too conservative and that greater amounts of various vitamins are required to improve health, especially when we are ill. The fame of Nobelist Linus Pauling rests not only upon his profound discoveries in basic chemistry, but in his work with the relationship between vitamins and health. Pauling says that it is not enough to maintain merely the minimum recommended level of vitamins in our system.

Most people know that Pauling was an advocate of massive doses of vitamin C, not only for general maintenance of good health, but for actual prevention of heart disease and cancer. The book by Cameron and Pauling lays out the case, and includes a number of case histories that are provocative. Your time will not be wasted by reading this important book. The same can be said for the book by Ornish, also listed in the bibliography.

In early 1999 a combined study conducted by Fox Chase Cancer Center, Temple University, and Case Western Reserve University found that patients who regularly used antioxidants such as vitamins A, C, and E were one-third less likely to have mutations in their p53 genes.

As we age, we are more likely to fail to take in or produce the vital immune-boosting chemicals that we need. That is why it is necessary to add vitamin supplements to our diets, especially when we are ill. Proper daily levels of various vitamins for cancer patients are debated in the medical profession; no definitive large scale clinical data are available. Nevertheless, a number of statements can be made with some certainty:

Vitamin B complex is necessary.
Vitamin C is important.
Zinc plays a significant role in prostate health.
Selenium also plays an important role in prostate health.
Vitamin A is important.
Vitamin E is vital for many aspects of health.
Vitamin D seems to prevent microscopic tumors from spreading.
A number of **herbs**, such as garlic, and Siberian ginseng appear to be helpful.

Vitamin B Complex:

The B vitamins, especially B6, B12, and folate, are important to our bodies in many ways. These are usually found in red meat. For those on a vegetarian or vegan diet, this is a serious matter, as we may find ourselves short of the B complex. These people must be especially concerned that they receive enough B12. Vegans can suffer from this lack. Long term deficiencies of this vitamin can lead to serious health defects, not the least being early senile dementia. If you embrace a vegetarian diet be sure to take supplements of the vitamin B complex.

Vitamin C:

Vitamin C is an important anti-oxidant valuable for proper functioning of all our organs. It is doubtful that we normally consume enough fruits and vegetables to provide much more than the FDA minimum levels of this vitamin. Vitamin C is water-soluble. If we take more than the body can absorb during the day, it will be eliminated in our urine. For prostate cancer patients, many physicians recommend taking up to ten grams or more per day.

Zinc:

Laboratory tests prove that the element zinc is necessary for prostate health. But the amount must be regulated. The recommended daily intake is 15 to 50 milligrams of zinc per day. More than that can be dangerous, so do not overdose.

Selenium:

Selenium, too, is shown to be important. And, like zinc, one must not overdo selenium intake. Two hundred micrograms to 500 micrograms per day is often recommended. There is clinical evidence that zinc and selenium reduce prostate cancer death by as much as 50 percent. In men who have a high selenium level, prostate cancer is 50 percent lower than in men with lower levels of this element.

Vitamin A:

Vitamin A is an anti-oxidant that helps ward off infection. It helps regulate cell differentiation. Many parts of the developing world lack vitamin A in the diet, and poor health in the population can be traced to this deficiency.

Vitamin A is not water-soluble, so one must avoid too much of this vitamin. It can be toxic in large dosages. More than 25,000 IU's can result in hypervitaminosis A, a condition that must be avoided.

Vitamin D:

Recent clinical evidence suggests that a lack of vitamin D may increase the risk of prostate cancer. Men who reside in the far northern and far southern latitudes (where there is far less sunlight) seem to have a higher rate of prostate cancer. Experimental evidence shows that vitamin D possesses some properties that may inhibit tumor growth. Indeed, new studies suggest this nutrient has important potential for treating men with advanced cancer. Since oral dosage is difficult to assess, the sun provides a good way to cause vitamin D production by our bodies. Why not try fifteen minutes in the sun each day, shirtless or perhaps in shorts? (Remember, though, that if you suffer a " weight loss" as I do, to wear your hat to avoid skin cancer. And be sure to use a sunscreen). I usually spend an hour outdoors every day doing my yardwork and gardening chores.

If a regular dose of sunlight is not available where you live, many physicians recommend a daily oral intake of vitamin D of 400 IU to 800 IU.

Vitamin E:

We have more and more evidence that vitamin E plays an important role in combating prostate cancer. Earlier studies found no convincing evidence that this is so, but newer randomized studies indicate that men who took 50 IU of vitamin E daily for five to eight years had one third fewer cases of prostate cancer and about 40 percent fewer deaths from this cause.

Vitamin E is an important anti-oxidant, and many physicians recommend up to 800 IU per day. Vitamin E, working with selenium appears to give better anti-cancer results than either drug working alone. Studies now show that vitamin E assists in reducing the toxicity of a number of chemotherapy drugs. Beware of taking too much of this vitamin, however. Vitamin E is not water-soluble, so overdoses can accumulate in vital organs and become toxic.

West Virginia Medical School produced a randomized study of bladder cancer patients. Half of the patients were given massive doses of vitamins, while half were given the normal RDA supplements. After five years the cancer recurrence rate for those who took the large doses was less than half the rate of those who took the standard RDA doses.

If you are taking hormones, there are a number of downsides you must consider. Change in bone density is one of them. This condition can be remedied by taking a daily calcium supplement. This can be obtained at any drug store, and often it is formulated with an added component of vitamin D. There is some controversy regarding calcium and prostate cancer. Some believe that it *contributes* to cancer growth, so consult your physician before taking this supplement.

Your physician will monitor your liver function with regular blood tests while you are on hormones. Some men must delete various hormones if the blood tests indicate potential liver damage.

It is wise to discuss with your physicians what levels of vitamins you are taking or plan to take. There are some vitamins, such as vitamin A and vitamin E that can be harmful if taken in large doses. If you are preparing for surgery or radiation, be aware that the vitamins and herbs you take may interfere not only with the efficiency of the radiation treatment, but may also thin your blood. This can cause bleeding problems during and after surgery. In my case, I was asked to stop taking my vitamins several weeks prior to my seed implant procedure.

Herbs:

In addition to green tea, many physicians use garlic and Siberian ginseng herbs in their treatments. You should discuss these and other herbal possibilities with your physician before entering a concentrated vitamin or herbal dietary course. As with vitamins it is possible to overdo their use. Each individual will react differently to herbal combinations, as tolerances will vary. If you decide to include herbs in your diet, do so gradually and take note of any changes in your general health.

Beware the use of the popular saw palmetto herb to relieve urinary symptoms. This herb is often suggested to reduce urinary blockages and other symptoms of a swollen prostate. The danger here lies in a false sense of security if such symptoms are reduced. This may confuse the patient into thinking he is addressing BPH when he is really masking the fact that a cancer is present. Before utilizing herbal remedies for benign prostate and urinary conditions, be sure that you are cancer free. Be sure to drink large quantities of water along with your vitamins and herbs.

Remember This

We all know that proper vitamin balance is necessary for good health. The difficulty is that the medical profession is not clear about what exact levels of the various vitamins are required for normal health, let alone when illness, such as cancer, strikes. But we are in a fight and it makes sense to add a vitamin regimen to our daily nutrition. Review the literature on the subject and talk with your physicians about your conclusions.

You will probably be asked to stop taking vitamins for several weeks before surgery or radiation treatments.

Chapter 20

What About Exercise?

Exercise is required for health. We all know this. But how many of us lead lives in which exercise plays a significant role? Should we not include exercise in our daily routines as a matter of course? Studies of the elderly show that even a minimal daily exercise program contributes to longevity. Participating in aerobic exercises or lifting some light hand weights brings measurable improvements. Not all of us need to go to the extent of a 92-year-old woman I read about, who is working on her black belt in karate, but the lesson is clear: Exercise is important to good health and a long life.

Evidence mounts that regular exercise is beneficial in the fight against cancer of *all* kinds. Exercise releases endocrines into the body, provides a sense of accomplishment and tones the body. A good, regular, exercise program will improve your immune system for the fight ahead.

Studies at the Loma Linda University in California show that even moderate exercise has many very positive effects. Exercise increases levels of interleukin-1, a protein that stimulates the activity of T cells. Moderate exercise can increase longevity. Elderly people who exercise daily show less incidence of cardiovascular disease, and they are less apt to die of cancer. Researchers show, however, that over-exercise is detrimental. Colds and respiratory infections actually increase in those who exercise too much. A reasonable balance must be found that benefits you.

Dr. Thomas Tomasi, at the Roswell Park Cancer Institute in Buffalo, New York, has presented evidence that relatively low levels of regular exercise reduced cardiovascular disease, and patients under study were less likely to die of cancer. In a large study of Seventh-Day Adventist men, obese men had significantly increased risk of death from prostate cancer, compared to men who were within their recommended weight range.

Start with breathing exercises. Take a dozen deep breaths and on the last breath, force every bit of air from your lungs. The next breath in will be very filling. Do this several times during the day.

Stretch your legs while standing and seated. When you are seated on the edge of a hard chair place your legs straight with your heels on the floor. If you slide your hands along your outstretched legs, trying to touch your toes, you will find that your lower back limbers up. Your legs will enjoy the stretch, too. Do this in a rocking fashion, each time reaching a bit further.

Do some knee bends by holding onto the back of a chair. Bend as deeply as you feel comfortable in doing. Do this several dozen times, perhaps a few times a day.

If you have a cycle machine, use it. Your thighs will register the exercise and you can build up some lung stamina, too.

Develop a brisk walking program. Walk every day to the point that your heart and lungs get a decent workout. If you can, walk with a partner, lover, or family member.

Develop exercise skills that will build strength, endurance, flexibility, and balance. These will help you lose weight, decrease blood pressure and heart rate, and reduce the potential for falls and related injury.

Do some stomach exercises, sit-ups and torso stretches. Or purchase an inexpensive tummy exercise device and develop "washboard abs." Even if you have a weak back you will find these are wonderful devices to strengthen your tummy muscles, and in such a way that low back discomfort is less a problem. Tone those stomach muscles so that your surgeon is impressed, and so that your recovery is made smoother.

Try a few minutes each day doing arm exercises with five-pound hand weights. You can do these while watching the evening news, for instance. You can also do a modified pushup routine, but with your body resting on your knees while you are in a kneeling position.

Do everything in your power to prepare your body for either surgery or for radiation of some kind. Even if you choose watchful waiting or hormone treatment, a healthy body will assist you in many ways. Improve your physician's track record by your personal commitment to a healthy, firm, active body.

What have you got to lose, except maybe a few unwanted pounds?

Finally, do your Kegel exercises (exercises designed to strengthen your urinary sphincter muscles) to make sure that your urinary control ability is maximized and in shape *before* your treatment. Whether or not you choose surgery or radiation you will want the strongest urinary sphincter muscles possible. Post-treatment results clearly show that those who have tight sphincters and good control of them before treatment have less incontinence after treatment. And, as you age, you will want to maintain your Kegel abilities for the rest of your life. They are very simple to learn and use.

The book by Bostwick titled *Prostate Cancer*, listed in the bibliography, provides a routine to follow. Remember you can do these exercises under all sorts of conditions: Standing up, in your office chair, while driving the car. Plan your Kegel work so that it comes almost automatically to you. Be aware at all times of the day that a few minutes here and there will work wonders for you. As bothersome as this is, you will be repaid a thousand times over by these simple exercises. Brief Kegel exercise instructions are found in Appendix G.

Remember This

If you went through the military experience, you were first sent to boot camp. This was to prepare you as fully as possible for battle. With cancer, you again are going into

battle. You need to prepare yourself both mentally and physically to defeat your new enemy.

A regular exercise routine will not only benefit your heart and body, but also your mind. Part of your preparation for successful therapy is to reduce stress as much as possible. Exercise plays an important role in stress management.

Chapter 21

Attitude and Work

I know of a man who, upon learning he had prostate cancer, immediately sold all his property and prepared for the end. This shows a profoundly negative attitude, most likely based on ignorance, coupled with unreasoned fear.

Prostate cancer is fraught with such emotional overtones that many men psychologically shut the subject out of their minds, hoping that it will go away, or they do not wish to explore the subject in depth as it is too frightening. This attitude can be a fatal error. I believe that the best course is to learn all you can about the subject, and if cancer does appear, be prepared to deal with it effectively.

Men who contract cancer of any kind have a psychologically-induced lowered libido. It is as if the mere *thought* of having cancer prevents men from engaging in sex. When cancer strikes one's prostate, the center of maleness, the emotions can be impacted very powerfully. But, you are not alone in all this. Your condition will concern your wife, family, and friends. Your sexuality and emotions are part of your wife's life too, and it is important to retain intimacy. This will have a material result by improving your treatment outcome. Remember while you are going through this that it is vital to let those around you know your emotional state as well as your physical condition.

From the beginning of this guide I have advocated the maintenance of a positive attitude, brought about by research, study, and education. Combine this with increased physical activity and the preparation of your Treatment Option Decision Charts and physician questionnaires, and you *will* develop a positive attitude, quite the opposite of the negative attitude demonstrated by the ignorant and fearful man.

"Resilience" is the ability to get through difficult or stressful times and overcome adversity. The National Cancer Institute recently urged more study of resilient cancer patients, those who survive terrible odds. It is hoped that the traits shown by these patients can be identified so that all of us can generate added strengths to combat illness. The most resilient people show a "learning" reaction to disturbing news and do not assume the role of a victim. I urge you to adopt a positive psychology, one that builds on your strengths, your relationships and your new knowledge of prostate cancer.

Most men are often impatient and uneasy dealing with medical problems of any kind. During my treatments I met many men who were in almost total ignorance of the broader issues of what was happening to them and what the future would hold for them. I sensed that these men were fearful of what was happening to them and lacked that faculty of "resilience." My feeling was these men were entering therapy with two strikes against them.

Women tend to be more pro-active in health matters, asking more questions of their physicians. And women see physicians some 27 percent more often than men do, according to an industry consultant. We should emulate women more closely, asking about everything; prognosis, treatment options, side effects, and how the remainder of our lives will be affected by the decisions we make at this stage of discovery. You do not want to be a victim, nor do you want to be fatalistic. Nor do you want to make a snap decision with regard to treatment. Find out the basics, as I have suggested throughout this guide, then resolve to work your way calmly through the decision process.

Appendix E provides a list of questions that might be appropriate for a dialogue with your physician. You will surely add to this list as you prepare for treatment. Do not be shy in asking any question. This is no time to be reticent.

After you have begun your research, continue working as before. Focus on your tasks at work and prepare to be even more productive than you normally are.

In your spare time, paint the bedroom, panel that clothes

closet with cedar as you have long intended doing. Tear up that worn kitchen vinyl flooring and replace it. You have long planned to do this, so do it now.

You will find that your mind will process ideas about your medical condition on its own, now that you have sensitized and prepared it. All sorts of ideas will float up to your consciousness while you are laying that kitchen floor. In physical work you will find a well-spring of ideas with which to attack your medical situation. Count on it!

Howard Greenwald, in his book *Who Survives Cancer*, makes many provocative points. He found, for instance, that there are personality traits and economic/social conditions that favor survival of cancer of any kind. These include education and higher economic status. Wealthier and more educated individuals have better diet and health attitudes than the general public. This is partly because this segment of society also has regular medical examinations, and early detection during a routine and regular medical exam often finds cancer of all kinds at its earliest detectable stage.

Greenwald stresses that early detection is essential for the best survival rates, and that survival depends upon advanced technology, as well as patient attitude and education about health matters. "Early detection has a real and meaningful effect on survival."

Remember This

Your knowledge about your condition and your attitude about it will have profound effects on the success of your treatment. The medical literature is filled with accounts of patients with positive attitudes who have overcome serious, even "hopeless" illness.

Be open with your physician. Shyness is not an admirable trait here. He needs to know your worries and fears. You should show him that you have taken the time to

educate yourself, that you have a positive attitude and that you and he will succeed.

Chapter 22

Chemotherapy, Alternative, and Clinical Trial Therapies

Garnick states that hormone therapy, outlined in Chapter 17, "is not a form of traditional cancer chemotherapy, as many patients initially believe." The purpose of hormone treatment is to block the male hormones that are required for a tumor to grow. In contrast, chemotherapy uses potent drugs that attempt to seek out and poison tumor cells.

At the present time there are no known drug treatments that can completely cure prostate cancer. Most drugs are used as a palliative, meaning they make one as comfortable as possible under the circumstances. They are for men with high-stage cancer.

In recent years a great deal of research has been directed to "alternative" treatments, meaning therapies that are outside the traditional surgical and radiation procedures. With greater public awareness of prostate cancer, the pace of such research will continue to accelerate. There are a number of encouraging avenues on the horizon. These include:

Purely **chemical approaches**
Herbal studies

Three other promising areas of research are covered in Chapter 24. They are vaccine development, genetic engineering approaches and anti-angiogenesis, or blood vessel-blocking chemicals.

Chemical Approaches:

We have all heard about chemotherapy being used for other types of cancer. Perhaps we know friends who have undergone such treatments and have observed the difficulties they endured. The use of chemotherapy for prostate therapy has not been well-established, because prostate cancer and a few other cancers, such as melanoma, are usually chemically resistant from the very start. As yet, chemotherapy drugs do not attack cancer cells with great precision and are rather toxic to normal cell tissue as well. Often, during drug treatments, the cancer cells develop further mutations that make them even *more* resistant to drugs. This is because the unstable tumor DNA mutates further as the cells divide. The DNA accumulates mutations that make them even more impervious to chemotherapeutic approaches.

The drug resistance of prostate cancer is one of the many factors that has made the development of anti-cancer drugs so difficult. So far, traditional chemotherapies have been shown to be ineffective in early diagnosed cancer of the prostate. Chemotherapy is usually used for advanced cases of prostate cancer, after cancer has spread to other sites in the body, and after hormone therapy has failed.

Many doctors are more familiar with chemotherapy treatments than with the newer hormonal approaches, and chemotherapy offers a greater profit to the physician than does hormone treatment. For the patient, however, the best quality of life is usually associated with the less toxic hormone therapy, if it first proves effective in reducing one's PSA.

Drugs have the advantage of being systemic, which means that they can attack cancer cells in all their forms and locations. It does not mean that all cancer cells can be eliminated by a single chemotherapy drug. This is why combinations of drugs are used.

Chemotherapy drugs are less effective on large tumor masses. In fact, chemotherapy is often employed after the main tumor has been removed or irradiated.

Many chemical drugs are being used for advanced cases, and drugs are coming on line that are, as yet, regarded as experimental. Scientists are conducting many clinical trials to find out the cancer-killing effects of a number of promising drugs. If your cancer has metastasized, your physician will no doubt recommend trial drugs for your condition. The book by Bostwick, listed in the bibliography and titled *Prostate Cancer,* has a chapter on chemotherapy that is a good starting point for your investigations. The book by Morra and Potts titled *The Prostate Cancer Answer Book,* also listed in the bibliography, provides additional information regarding alternative therapies and clinical trials. The book by Drs. Lewis and Berger discusses the subject and describes a number of interesting clinical trials.

Just because such chemicals are available does not mean they are fully effective. Clinics are attempting to learn how effective these compounds are. You may wish, in consultation with your physician, to participate in a clinical trial for a chemotherapy approach. Many recognized and legitimate cancer centers across the nation offer programs for various therapeutic approaches. The book by Drs. Bostwick, MacLennan, and Larson, cited in the bibliography, has a discussion on a number of such possibilities.

We ought not to despair because of the slow pace or lack of dramatic clinical success in this field. Progress is being made, slow as it is. After all, the breakthrough in breast cancer with the advent of tamoxifen came after years of research and testing among tens of thousands of women. Even so, not all patients are cured by this drug.

Marks points out that a compound called spermine that is naturally manufactured by the prostate seems to inhibit prostate cancer growth. This may explain why cancer growth in its early stages is slow, while growth is rapid once the tumor material has escaped from the prostate. At the present time there is no medication based on spermine, but considerable investigation is being done in this field.

In your studies you may run across the word "cytokine." Cytokines are naturally occurring compounds that have a killing effect on cancer, because they prompt T cells to proliferate. It is hoped that a cytokine gene may be transferred into tumor cells, thereby promoting an immune attack upon the cancer. A great deal of research is being done in this area, and clinical trials are now in progress on vaccines for pancreatic and prostate cancer at the Johns Hopkins University Medical School. Here, the specific patient's tumor material is combined with a cytokine gene and released back into the tumor. It is hoped that this approach will cause the immune system to attack every cell that contains this marker. A success would bring a strong immunotherapeutic approach for all prostate cancer patients.

Herbal Approaches:

While it is undeniable that many herbs can help in the fight, there is little evidence that herbal treatment by itself is effective in eliminating cancer. But, as part of an improved diet, herbs ought to be considered in your treatment as immune system boosters. Indeed, of the body's various systems, none is more receptive to herbal assistance than the immune system. Herbs may be useful in strengthening the activity of the T cells, energizing our macrophages, and in suppressing cancer cell production.

One promising herbal blend is called PC SPES, a blend of eight herbs that physicians believe can help in the fight. Validation studies for this herbal mixture are still required. Considerable anecdotal evidence suggests that many patients are helped by this treatment and that this combination of herbs can kill tumor cells that no longer respond to hormonal control. Many physicians are prescribing this herbal blend. The herbs chosen for this blend are divided into five categories as follows:

Immune-stimulating
Anti-tumor activity
Anti-viral activity
Anti-inflammatory properties

Anti-benign prostate hyperplasia properties

We are advised not to depend upon this supplement alone, but we hope it will prevent or delay recurrence of prostate cancer, lengthen survival time for patients, improve effectiveness of conventional treatments, delay the requirement for more powerful chemotherapy, shrink the tumor, and perhaps eliminate the need for hormone therapy. You may wish to discuss this subject with your physician and to consult a number of books in the bibliography that contain essays on herbs as adjunct treatment.

In the meantime, beware of any "treatment" that is advertised or touted as being in some way "special" or "ignored," or "shunned" by medical science. Medical science is so active, with so many physicians looking for new treatments and with so many investigations going on, that it is quite doubtful that some effective and powerful "unknown" treatment could or would be on the market. If it sounds too good to be true, it ought to be regarded with suspicion.

You will find references to a diet called "macrobiotic," meaning a diet consisting primarily of cereal products and rice, and without meat, animal products, sugar, or milk products. More and more evidence is accumulating that reduction or avoidance of the latter can help. Dr. James P. Carter, a professor at Tulane School of Public Health says that prostate cancer "tops the list" of cancers that can respond dramatically to a macrobiotic diet. Some patients can experience an amazing turnaround in their condition.

A diet leaning toward Chinese cuisine is often a valuable adjunct to whatever therapy you are undertaking. I know of a prostate cancer patient, otherwise in good health and physically active, who cut his PSA in half merely by adhering to Chinese cuisine, giving up all alcoholic beverages and soft drinks containing sugar.

You should also consider your lifestyle as part of your therapy. Do you eat too many foods that are identified with prostate cancer? Do you maintain a high stress job or lifestyle? Do you drink more than is recommended? Can you truly relax regularly? Dr. Dean Ornish of the Preventive Medicine Research Institute in Sausalito, California, achieved fame a decade ago with his research into the effects that life style and diet exert on our hearts. He now has five-year data supporting an ultra-low-fat diet, combined with exercise. He shows how this can reduce cholesterol deposits in our arteries. His results show a 50 percent reduction of "cardiac events" for those in the study.

Ornish is now working with prostate cancer patients and is heading up a provocative program with the UCSF Medical Center in San Francisco. This program concentrates on lifestyle, yoga, diet, and group therapy to see if these factors have as much effect on preventing or removing prostate cancer as they seem to have in improving the condition of our hearts.

If you require chemotherapy or are in clinical trials of some kind, most likely your general health is the controlling factor in your life. Physical disruptions to your life from these treatments are less than is the case of the invasive therapies. Your schedules will be governed by the routine established by the chemotherapy procedures and your reactions to the treatment.

Remember This

It is understandable that we all hope that we can escape our dilemma with non-invasive therapies in place of surgery or radiation. While on-going research provides promise for the future, we must not bet our lives that such help will arrive before our condition escapes the window of opportunity allowed for standard treatment. Such a bet entails enormous risk, and cannot be recommended at this time.

Chapter 23

Imaging

The Japanese ideogram for photography is "seeing the truth." Your physicians will want to "see the truth" for several reasons, and they will employ a number of sophisticated imaging devices beyond mere X-rays. You will want to see the truth too, as this will help you know your enemy and visualize it. This will help you in your combat.

Your physician will use these methods as diagnostic tools to identify and locate your tumors. He also needs them to define treatment parameters, especially if you choose radiation of some kind.

Your doctor will want to know exactly where your tumors are, whether they are truly confined within the prostate, are about to break out of the capsule wall, or if they have already done so. If one has, the doctor will want to know where extra-capsular tumors have taken root, whether cancer cells have entered your seminal vesicles, nearby lymph nodes, or, in rare cases, if cancer tumors have metastasized at distant locations, such as your hips, ribs, spine, or liver.

Your physicians will use a number of devices to make their determinations:

X-rays
Sonograms
CAT scans
MRI

X-rays:

Using X-ray photography, your doctor will be able to learn the basic layout of your pelvic region. While this photography does not discriminate between tumor and normal tissue, X-rays will help a surgeon when he makes his incision. X-rays will show your pubic bone, the location and shape of which is also a significant factor in planning any radiation treatment. Accurate X-rays will be required when your radiologist configures the computer program that will ultimately direct the radiation to your prostate.

Sonograms:

Your first exposure to a sonogram will probably be when needle biopsies are taken. This examination is a bit more invasive than mere X-rays, but it is not painful. The trans-rectal ultrasound transducer is inserted in your rectum and the sound waves that penetrate your prostate and surrounding tissue will give your physician an accurate image on a television screen. From here he can locate any suspicious areas within your prostate.

Then he will be able to direct thin needles to those areas to obtain minute tissue samples which will be sent to the pathology laboratory. This sonogram procedure will also give him valuable information about the shape of your prostate, the volume of your prostate and the volume of the tumor.

If you choose seed implantation treatment you will have a second session with the sonogram, but this time you will be unconscious. The radiologist will image your prostate with sonography and monitor the accurate placement of the radioactive seeds while he is inserting them. In this way he can be sure that each seed is being placed exactly where the computer program has calculated to distribute them.

CAT scans:

The CAT scan (computer-assisted tomography) imaging system will be used if you are to receive radiation treatments. Coupled with X-ray imagery, a three-dimensional mathematical model of your prostate will be placed in a computer, and from this model, all the focussing instructions are automatically calculated for the external beams that will send the killing radiation into your prostate.

MRI:

Magnetic resonance images are generated by a very noisy machine that is the least invasive method to obtain images of your body. The magnetic resonance imaging system places your pelvic area under strong magnetic fields. These magnetic fields slightly disrupt molecules within your body. When the field is turned off the molecules return to their normal state, and it is at this time that the computer records the different responses that various tissues make. A photograph can then be made of these differences.

Combining magnetic spectroscopic imaging with the endorectal coil MRI is an exciting new development of MRI imaging, employed by the UCSF Medical Center in San Francisco, and at Memorial Sloan-Kettering Medical Center in New York City. A probe containing a coil that emits radiofrequency waves is inserted into the rectum and rests against the prostate. This procedure is no more uncomfortable than the standard sonogram procedure. The results of this combined technique are fine quality photographs of your prostate, seminal vesicles, bladder, rectum, and urethra. The results are superior to ultrasound techniques and are quite accurate in discriminating between healthy tissue and tumor material. It is hoped that within the next few years, many other clinics across the nation will be able to offer this accurate and valuable technique.

This technique can provide a high level of confidence for determining the location, volume, and possible extracapsular spread of tumor material.

New machines are increasing the accuracy and diagnostic ability of your physician to "see" your tumor no matter where it may be. All of these techniques are very potent tools for your doctor. It is of critical importance to obtain the most detailed picture of your situation. No matter what treatment technique you ultimately decide upon, the more accurate a picture your physician has, the more successful he will be.

And, the images are important to you on a personal level. Seeing your enemy will energize you and give you confidence that it surely *has* been located and is not some theoretical medical figment.

Remember This

Do not be deterred for any reason from obtaining images of your prostate with the devices mentioned here. Your physician must have them to increase his success. I urge each patient to see as many images of his condition as possible and discuss them with his physician. Your confidence will be raised, and so will the potential for your successful treatment.

Employing a combination of these diagnostic techniques will aid in determining the most effective treatment for you. The results of these images ought to be an integral part of the treatment decision process for you and your physicians.

Finally, these imaging techniques will have an important role in the years after treatment. They will provide an objective validation to correlate with the results of your PSA testing.

Chapter 24

What the Future May Hold

We all have read or heard that despite major advances in the cure for leukemia, there has been very little improvement in other cancer statistics over the past two decades or more. But in the case of early-detected prostate cancer, our treatment options *do* give us reason to cheer. Early detected cancer of the prostate *can* be cured, with a very high success rate. The new techniques now available allow very accurate surgery, radiation, seed implants and cryosurgery, all of which yield impressive statistics. For a man aged 60 or above, these statistics approach the life expectancy numbers he could count on if he were unaffected by cancer at all.

A great deal of work is being done outside the traditional surgical and radiation fields. Major and important clinical experimental programs are available to test many promising treatments.

The principal arenas of new research are:

Vaccine development
Genetic engineering approaches
Anti-angiogenesis chemicals that prevent blood vessel development to the tumor

Vaccines:

Active cancer tumors somehow manage to sidestep or short-circuit the natural immune system responses to their presence. Otherwise, they would not have been allowed by the body to grow into threatening tumors.

In a sense the immune system is reluctant to attack tumor cells because it cannot attack its own tissue. Since tumor material was derived from normal prostate cells, our body's auto-immune response is tricked.

The goal of a "therapeutic" vaccine is to prod the body to cure itself with its own, perhaps weakened or tricked, immune system. Effective vaccines will allow our bodies to recognize and attack prostate cancer cells anywhere in the body, while leaving normal cells alone. Such a vaccine could act not only as a preventative, but it would also be valuable for men who have already undergone treatment of some kind. New vaccines for many conditions are being prepared and readied for market, as there have been many "proof-of-principle" experiments. The discovery of T cell-specific antigens is going to revolutionize cancer immunology studies. A great deal of medical research and development is going into this promising field, and research laboratories around the world are putting large amounts of money into the effort. The financial rewards for successful vaccines will be enormous.

A successful vaccine for prostate cancer will most likely be made from fragments of an individual patient's tumor cells. Our immune system uses antibodies and T cells to identify and destroy infections, including cancer cells. Our bodies manufacture millions of them. They single out a specific target called an antigen.

Antigens are cell markers that the immune system uses to recognize what is a normal part of your body and what is abnormal or foreign to you. The term "antigen" indicates a molecule that triggers an immune response. Antibodies are proteins that recognize and attach to specific antigens. On injection, the antigens prepared from your cancer fragments will train your antibodies and killer T cells to recognize the cancer cells when they encounter them. The antibodies and T cells can then go to work destroying the tumor material anywhere it is found in your body.

An example of the immune stimulation approach is a new trial undertaken by the Department of Urology at UCLA, and the M.D. Anderson Cancer Center in Houston, using a technology developed by Northwest Biotherapeudics of Seattle. Four injections are composed of the patient's own purified immune stimulation cells, which have been removed and altered by a proprietary recombinant prostate specific membrane antigen. When the material is re-injected into the patient, his immune system is stimulated to search out and destroy tumor cells.

Dozens of large-scale controlled tests of cancer vaccines are underway in clinics around the world. If you want a list of clinical trials involving prostate cancer vaccines, contact the National Cancer Institute (800-4-CANCER, or at the internet address: www.cancernet.nci.nih.gov/pdq) There is also a major focus on melanoma, the fast-growing skin cancer that strikes about one percent of us. The first melanoma vaccine is now approved for use. This is a milestone event and promises future success in this exciting field.

Genetic Engineering:

Gene therapy is another avenue hotly pursued by research laboratories everywhere. No doubt it will take years before effective gene therapies are perfected, but, again, the financial rewards are so huge that a great deal of funding is being made available at this time.

Many areas of DNA research are being investigated in the fight against cancer. Monoclonal antibody studies (monoclonal antibodies are molecules engineered to seek and destroy cancer cells) are a promising arena of investigation. The ultimate goal of these gene researchers is to tailor-make drugs specifically for each cancer patient. It may be that there are as many different cancers as there are patients. Tailor-made drugs would not target prostate cancer or breast, lung, or liver cancer, but the specific errant gene that the individual may carry within his own tumor. Scientists hope gene therapies will allow the creation of a tumor cell that is made killable. Altered gene fragments, for instance, could be introduced into a cancer cell where they will either normalize the cancer cell's activity or accelerate its death. A great deal of research work is being done in this field, and hope is high.

Other research focuses on chemicals that could be injected or fed into the blood stream. The drug would arrive only at cells that produce PSA, ignoring all other cells. The drug would then program the PSA-producing cell to die. This cell-assisted suicide approach has promise. Testing will begin soon.

Each tumor is unique: It has its own particular derangement of DNA. One of the most common indicators of DNA derangement concerns the gene labeled p53. This gene is a "cell protector" gene. In normal cells this gene attempts to prevent mutations and tries to repair the cell if a mutation appears. It seems to be a growth regulator gene and may also cause self-destruction by apoptosis (the medical term for genetically programmed cell death) of unstable cells. Some mutations can inactivate this gene. When this happens, cancer tumors mutate much more rapidly than if this gene is not damaged. It appears that cancer cells are no longer subject to apoptosis, hence they may be immortal. When we have a damaged p53 gene, our tumors become resistant to hormonal treatments and chemotherapy. A mutated p53 gene was associated with a 20-to-30-fold increased risk of death by prostate cancer. So an altered p53 gene is a very important measurement. This factor may be part of the statistics associated with aneuploid tumor cells. Detailed biopsy studies will help identify how dangerous your tumor type is.

Other genes are being discovered that, if damaged, may be involved in tumor production.

The goal of all this research, of course, is to find a "smart bomb" or a vaccine that can identify prostate cancer cells, search them out wherever they may be, and attach themselves to those cells and *only* those cells, excluding all normal cells. Once attached, the compound, whether it is a radioactive isotope, DNA or chemical agent, can deliver a toxin only to the cancer cells, sparing normal cells. We may be surprised how soon such devices will appear on the horizon. We will see them as useful, too, for patients who have already undergone surgery, radiation, or chemotherapy. They will be valuable in mopping up any stray cancer cells left over from the primary treatment.

Daily we see evidence of promise, not only for prostate cancer but for cancer of all kinds. The Pharmaceutical Research and Manufacturers of America, reporting in 1998, stated there are now more that 300 human cancer drug trials underway. This is indicative of the intense work being done on cancer drugs of all kinds.

An example of these promising therapies is an antibody drug that blocks a particular receptor on T cells. At the University of California at Berkeley and University Medical Center at San Francisco, plans are being made to conduct preliminary prostate cancer therapy trials. In animal experiments, melanoma and prostate cancer therapies have shown surprising results.

In this approach the T cell itself is altered so that its autoimmune "switch" is turned off. Rather than stimulating the T cell into more activity, the T cell will now recognize a tumor cell as foreign, where previously it believed it to be a normal body element.

The mice experiments were so encouraging that human clinical trials are to begin soon. One can easily see how important a breakthrough will be for patients with metastatic cancer, where sites may exist in many locations in the body.

In the mice experiments for melanoma, the mice were immune to a subsequent injection of melanoma cells. This result is highly suggestive that the therapy is not only curative, but protective as well.

Anti-angiogenesis:

In 1998 very encouraging test results were released regarding Dr. Judah Folkman's tumor strangulation discoveries.

Cancer tumors emit specific growth chemicals (angiogenic factors) that stimulate the body to develop blood vessels to support the tumor. Once an incipient tumor reaches a certain size it must obtain nourishment from the body in order to grow, and an adequate blood supply is required. In 1998, EntreMed, Inc. burst into public view with sensational test results for angiostatin and endostatin, chemicals that reduced or removed cancer in mice by cutting off the tumor's blood supply. These chemicals block the signals that are sent out to build blood vessels to the tumor. Human tests began in 1999. The laboratory tests indicate that the use of endostatin when combined with radiation may be more effective than radiation alone.

Some 25 companies are currently working on anti-angiogenesis drugs. It is easy to imagine how financially important a workable anti-angiogenesis drug could be to a modern bio-tech company. This field is one of the most active areas of cancer research.

Folkman's work has been going on for years, during which he has endured serious professional skepticism by many who have suggested that his research is too far off the mainstream. Folkman felt that if drugs could be created to cut off a tumor's ability to persuade blood vessels to develop a blood supply to the tumor (which also later acts as the avenue the tumor uses to spread to other parts of the body), the tumor would be starved of nutrients and die. The word "angiogenesis," refers to the formation of new blood vessels in an organism. Folkman's work is a search for anti-angiogenesis drugs, drugs that have already produced tumor death in mice. This field holds great promise for treatment for all human cancers. An encouraging side role for endostatin is in heart disease. Recent tests suggest that endostatin prevents blood vessel development to the fatty deposits that build up in our arteries. We could see this therapy used for heart patients as well as for cancer patients.

Folkman is quick to point out, however, that years of testing will be required before we know whether it will work in humans. Even if such drugs *are* applicable, Folkman sees them not as a cure for cancer, but as an adjunct to other treatments such as chemotherapy, radiation, gene, and vaccine therapies. He thinks anti-angiogenesis drugs will not replace the standard treatments now used to treat prostate cancer. His drugs are really an end run around the fact that unstable tumor cells ultimately become drug-resistant.

It is wise for us to remember that it was only four decades or so ago that Watson and Crick unraveled the structure of DNA, the basic building block of life. Much has happened since that discovery to increase our knowledge of how life works. Amazingly, it appears that scientists soon will completely decipher the human genome, perhaps within two years! We must not allow ourselves to turn our backs on the wonderful promise that resides in this research. Scientists are already curing many genetic defects in humans by manipulating their basic DNA chemistry. Many more cures and treatments are in the pipeline as the century turns.

So many approaches to the cure for prostate cancer are being announced that there appears to be an "epidemic" of such news. The pace is very rapid. Can anyone think that DNA treatments for cancer of all kinds can be very far off?

Remember This

For those of us living in Europe and America, the greatest gift of the century is the extension of life span. Improvements in living conditions, coupled with amazing advances in medicine, have improved and extended life beyond what might have been imagined when the century began.

As we enter a new century, new technologies certainly represent the wave of the future. Unfortunately, those of us recently diagnosed cannot sit and wait, like the hapless men waiting for Godot, putting off decisions and action, hoping to be saved by some form of new technology. We have to do something now.

As exciting as the new prospects are, a significant number of techniques mentioned in the press will probably not pan out. It may be tantalizing or tempting to wait for such technologies as a primary treatment option, but there are dangers in waiting, especially for those who are still in the window of opportunity where it is wise to decide among the treatment options open now. The future technologies, for now, must remain just that...future potential options, perhaps available as secondary options in case primary treatment fails.

Chapter 25

Dealing With Negative Thoughts

When dark moods descend upon you, turn to your Treatment Option Decision Charts and Future Treatment Trade-off Charts for support. Consult them to remind yourself that you *do* have a handle on the situation. This will have a powerful effect upon your emotions.

Remember, you are not helpless. You have a brain, and you have information on which to decide and act. You have a desire to become well. So, do not allow your condition to make you feel helpless or hopeless.

Keep a running list of questions to pose to your physicians, a *written* list. This will give you a sense of empowerment. Both of these exercises will relieve anxieties and aid your physician in treating you. You may discover that the outcome of whatever treatment you choose will be *better* than you imagined along the way.

Take long walks with a loved one. Listen to music. Concentrate on those spiritual aspects of your life that have brought you pleasure and strength in times of past difficulties.

Think about this when you are depressed: Suppose your primary treatment is surgery or radiation of some kind that ultimately fails to remove all of the cancer. The treatment bought you several years of life, and you have avenues open to you to buy more. If you have surgery that ultimately fails, then you turn to radiation. This will add several more years of life even in the event that this, too, fails to cure you.

With the failed cases, you still have cryosurgery to look into, or hormone treatments of some kind. Now you are a decade along the line, and during this time incredible amounts of money and genius will have been expended to find DNA or vaccine approaches to control prostate cancer. No doubt by the time you exhaust all the treatment possibilities you will be older than 75 or 80 and concerned with *other* health matters. The coming DNA and vaccine technologies will let you concentrate on the other issues of aging with a free mind and the knowledge that you have managed your condition very well indeed.

Remember This

Unless your cancer is in a state of advanced metastasis, you are in a position to control the situation and your health. You have many treatment options before you and many opportunities to work toward keeping cancer in remission after your treatment. Time is on your side, and you should organize your life so you will be in control of your future.

Chapter 26

Loose Ends

You will not eliminate the subject of cancer from your life. The periodic PSA tests will serve as a constant reminder to maintain vigilance. If you prepare your body, you will appear for your treatment with many advantages. If you prepare your mind for a thoughtful and reasoned tradeoff decision process, you will discover that if you are among the fortunate *majority* of men, you *will* eliminate cancer from your body.

We all are beset with that aspect of living that seems to run against us—time, that almost mythical concept that seems to pass at ever-faster rates as we age. It gets worse as we grow older, and we live with the feeling that we have barely a moment to spare from an overcrowded agenda of tasks before us. Where does time "go" when it goes? And where is Einstein when we need him to help us with this question?

I will close this guide with a quote from Maurice Goudeket, the 19th century author of *The Delights of Growing Old*, a quote that may help us all explore more fully what remains of the time left to us:

Every fresh day finds me more filled with wonder and better qualified to draw the last drop of delight from it.

Think about it.

Remember This

I mentioned in my acknowledgments at the very beginning of this book that my experience with prostate cancer has rewarded me with a "truly life-enhancing experience."

Perhaps contracting prostate cancer should be viewed as a wake-up call, a summons that, if we respond, can motivate us to fulfill our destinies to live life to the fullest.

Bibliography

This is a list of recommended books to read for general background prostate information and discussion of the various treatments available.

Details of the various treatments that you can choose from can be obtained easily in any bookstore or library. The books cited provide further background information for prostate cancer treatment procedures, and these books are recommended reading. The books by Dr. Sheldon Marks, Dr. David Bostwick, Dr. Marc Garnick, and Marion Morra and Eve Potts, are inexpensive and easily obtainable in your public library or at your local bookstore. Information on prostate cancer and cancer research expands monthly.

Bostwick, David G. — ***Prostate Cancer: What Every Man and his Family Needs to Know.*** Villard, 1996

Cameron, Ewan & Pauling, Linus — ***Cancer and Vitamin C.*** Camino Books, 1993

Consumer Reports — "Herbal Roulette."***Consumer Reports Study*** on Herbal Remedies for Many Health Issues. Nov. 1995

Kaltenback, Don — ***Prostate Cancer: A Survivor's Guide.*** Seneca House Press,1995

Garnick, Marc B. — ***The Patient's Guide to Prostate Cancer.*** Plume Books, 1996

Garnick, Marc B. & Fair, William R. — "Prostate Cancer." ***Scientific American,*** December, 1998

Greenfield, Louise	***Cancer Overcome by Diet: An Alternative to Surgery.*** Self-published, Livorna, Mich., 1995
Greenwald, H.	***Who Survives Cancer?*** Univ. of California Press, 1992
Lewis, J., & Berger, E.	***New Guidelines for Surviving Prostate Cancer*** Health Education Publisher, 1997
Lewis, J.	***Best Options for Diagnosing and Treating Prostate Cancer.*** Health Education Publisher, 1999
Margolis, S. & Carter, H.B.	***Prostate Disorders 1997*** Johns Hopkins White Paper
Marks, Sheldon	***Prostate And Cancer: A Family Guide to Diagnosis, Treatment, and Survival.*** Fisher Books, 1995
Medina, John	***The Clock of Ages.*** Cambridge University Press, 1996
Milken, Michael	***Taste for Living Cookbook*** Time-Life Books, 1998
Morra, M. & Potts, E.	***The Prostate Cancer Answer Book*** Avon Books, 1996
Pilgrim, Aubrey	***A Revolutionary Approach to Prostate Cancer.***

	Sterling House Publishers, 1998
Ornish, Dean	***Reversing Heart Disease.*** Ballantine Books, 1991
Ornish, Dean	***Love and Survival.*** Harper Collins, 1998
Rosenfeld, Isadore	***Guide to Alternate Medicine.*** Random House, 1996
Sattilaro, Anthony	***Living Well Naturally.*** Houghton Mifflin, 1984
Stamey, Thomas A.	***1997 Monographs in Urology***, vol 18, #6.

These are additional scientific papers you might obtain from the library, the Internet, or from your physicians.

Blaese, R. Michael	"Gene Therapy for Cancer." ***Scientific American,*** June 1997
Blasko, J., Wallner, K., et al.	"Prostate Specific Antigen Based Disease Control Following Ultrasound Guided 125 Iodine Implantation for Stage T1/T2 Prostatic Cancer." ***The Journal of Urology,*** vol. 154, 1995
Blasko, J., Ragde, H., et al.	"Should Brachytherapy Be Considered a Therapeutic Option in Localized Prostate Cancer?" ***The Urologic Clinics of North America,*** vol. 23, #4, 1996

Garnick, Marc B. "The Dilemmas of Prostate Cancer." ***Scientific American,*** April 1994

Grimm, P., Blasko, J., et al. "Does Brachytherapy have a Role in the Treatment of Prostate Cancer?" **Hematology/Oncology Clinics of America**, vol. 10, #3, 1996

Grove, Andy "Taking on Prostate Cancer." ***Fortune Magazine,*** 13 May 1996

Harris, Louis "Perspectives on Prostate Cancer Treatments: Awareness, Attitudes, and Relationships, 1995." Obtainable from ***US Too, International, Inc.***

Hanks, G. & Perez, C, et al. "PSA Confirmation of Cure at 10 Years of T1b, T2, M0 Prostate Cancer Patients Treated in RTOG Protocol 7706 with External Beam Irradiation." In the ***Journal of Radiation Oncology Biol. Phys.,*** vol 30,

McKay, J. & Hirano, N. ***The Chemotherapy and Radiation Therapy Survival Guide.*** New Harbinger Pub. 1998

Middleton, R. & Thompson, I. "Prostate Cancer Clinical Guidelines Panel Summary Report on the Management of Clinically Localized Prostate Cancer." ***The Journal of Urology,*** vol. 154, 1995

Myers, C, Myers, R.S, & Steck, S. ***Eating Your Way to Better Health.*** Rivanna Health Publication, 1999

Partin, A. et al. "Use of Prostate Specific Antigen, Clinical Stage and Gleason Score to Predict Pathological Stage in men with Localized Prostate Cancer." ***The Journal of Urology,*** vol. 150, 1993

Roach, M., Chinn, D., et al. "A Pilot Survey of Sexual Function and Quality of Life Following 3D Conformal Radiotherapy for Clinically Localized Prostate Cancer." ***Int. Journal of Radiation Oncology Biol. Phys.,*** vol 35 #5, 1996

Scientific American This issue of Scientific American is devoted entirely to discussions of new researches on cancer of all types, and is well worth the read. September, 1996

Varmus, H. & Weinberg, R. ***Genes and The Biology of Cancer.*** Scientific American Library, 1993

Yonemoto, L. & Slater, J. "Combined Proton and Photon Conformal Radiation Therapy for Locally Advanced Carcinoma of the Prostate." ***Int. Journal of Radiation Oncology Biol. Phys.,*** vol. 37, 1997

Zagars, G. "Radiotherapy for Clinically Localized Cancer of the Prostate." ***The Cancer Bulletin,*** vol. 45, #5, 1993

Appendix A

Glossary

The following is a short list of technical terms that you will encounter in your readings. It is not meant to be complete, but you should understand the meanings of these basic terms.

Adenocarcinoma: Cancer originating in a glandular tissue, such as the prostate.
Adjuvant therapy: Treatment used with or after a primary treatment. Hormone therapy often complements radiation or surgery, for instance.
Adrenal glands: Pair of organs located near the kidneys that secrete a number of important male hormones.
Agonist: Man-made drug that mimics the body's regulatory functions. Hormone therapy uses agonists that curtail the production of testosterone.
Alternative therapy: Treatment that does not rely upon surgery, radiation, or chemotherapy, but instead concentrates on diet, vitamins, exercise, and attitude to increase the body's immune system.
Androgen: Male hormones secreted by the testes and adrenal glands.
Aneuploid: A type of the ploidy of a cell showing an abnormal number of chromosomes.
Angiogenesis: Formation of new blood vessels to a tumor.
Anti-androgen: Drug used to counter the action of the androgens produced normally.
Anti-angiogenesis: Prevention of the formation of new blood vessels to a tumor.
Antibody: Naturally produced agents. The body produces antibodies that try to counteract the toxic effects of something that is foreign to the body, such as a disease.

Antigen: Substance that stimulates the body to produce antibodies.
Apoptosis: Programmed cell death. Cancer cells somehow avoid the built-in cell death regulators that normal cells have.
Benign prostatic hyperplasia (BPH): Non-cancerous enlargement of the prostate gland.
Benign tumor: Abnormal growth that is not a cancer and will not spread to other sites in the body.
Biopsy: Removal of a small amount of tissue for microscope examination for abnormal cells.
Bound-PSA: Prostate specific antigen in the blood that is bound to a protein molecule.
Brachytherapy: Radiation treatment for cancer that employs tiny radioactive metal "seeds," inserted into a tumor or very close to it.
CAT scan: Computer-generated cross-sections of X-ray images of the body used for diagnostic purposes.
Cancer: Abnormal growth that does not obey normal cellular controls, and thus can grow to invade and destroy other organs of the body and threaten life.
Capsule wall: Layer of cells forming the wall of the prostate gland.
Carcinogen: A substance that is known to induce cancer.
Chemotherapy: Use of powerful drugs to treat cancer.
Clinical trial: Research study that involves patients. Studies attempt to answer specific questions about health matters or new drugs.
Compromise: Term used to indicate potential lessening of health, or a possible reduction of effectiveness for a future treatment, if required.
Conformal: Treatment that conforms closely to the size and shape of your prostate and tumor.

Cryosurgery: Cryoablation or cryotherapy treatment for cancer that freezes tissue to kill cancer cells within that tissue.
Cystoscopy: An examination procedure in which the doctor looks into the urethra and bladder via a flexible light pipe.
Cytokine: A naturally occurring substance that has anti-tumor activity.
Digital Rectal Examination (DRE): Physician's examination of your prostate by insertion of his finger into your rectum to palpate the prostate.
Diploid: Ploidy of a cell containing the correct number of chromosomes.
DNA: Molecule that makes up genes.
Downsize: To reduce the volume of the prostate.
Downstage: To lower the stage assigned to a tumor as a result of some treatment, such as hormonal therapy.
DRE: See digital rectal examination.
Estrogen: A female sex hormone.
Extension: The possibility that tumor material has spread beyond the walls of the prostate.
External beam radiation: Radiation of an organ or tumor by a machine located outside the body, such as an X-ray generator.
Foley catheter: A small tube that drains the bladder, inserted through the urethra.
Free-PSA: Prostate specific antigen that is in the blood, but is not bound to any protein.
Gene: Basic unit of cellular life. Genes are inherited. Damage to a gene may influence erratic tumor growth.
Gland: Organ that secretes a fluid into or from the body.
Gleason grade: A classification system for the type of cancer cells that may be in the prostate.
Gleason score: A system used to determine the aggressive-

ness of tumor cells.

Godot: Central, but absent, character in a play (Waiting for Godot), by Samuel Beckett. Godot never appears.

Hormone: A chemical secreted by body organs that circulates and acts upon cells within the body.

Hormone therapy: Use of medicine that curtails the testosterone the body produces. Prostate cancer requires testosterone to grow, and this therapy prevents testosterone production.

Immune system: The body's natural system of defense against infection or foreign substances.

Implant: The tiny radioactive seeds that are employed in brachytherapy treatments.

Impotence: Loss of ability to sustain an erection.

Incontinence: Impairment of urinary control.

Interstitial radiation: Another name for brachytherapy.

Kegel exercise: Exercise to help strengthen the muscles that control urination.

Locally advanced prostate cancer: Term used to indicate that a tumor can be felt by the physician during the DRE. It does not necessarily mean that the patient has an advanced cancer condition.

Luteinizing hormone: A hormone that regulates the production of sex hormones in men.

Lycopene: Substance found in cooked tomatoes and other vegetables.

Lymphadenectomy: Removal of lymph nodes near the prostate to look for spread of cancer outside the prostate.

Lymph node: Filters for bacteria or cancer cells. Part of the lymphatic system.

Macrobiotic diet: A strict low-calorie vegetarian diet that may be helpful for treating cancer.

Malignant: Cancerous.

Metastasis: The spread of a cancer from its original site to another portion or organ of the body.

Morbidity: Unhealthy side effects resulting from a treatment procedure.

Mortality: Statistic of death.

MRI: Magnetic resonance imaging, using powerful magnetic fields to provide detailed images of the prostate.

Neoadjuvant: The practice of starting a patient on some protocol prior to the use of the primary therapy. A common example is the use of hormone drugs begun months before surgery or radiation is employed as primary treatment.

Oncologist: A physician who specializes in treating cancer patients.

Orchiectomy: Surgical removal of the testicles which is done to stop production of testosterone.

Organ-confined: The tumor is confined within the gland and has not escaped.

Palliation: Treatment to relieve symptoms and pain or discomfort, rather than to effect a cure.

Pathologist: Specialist who examines tissue samples or fluid from the body in order to diagnose disease.

Percutaneous suprapubic tube: A small urine drainage tube inserted into the bladder through the lower abdomen.

Ploidy: Analysis of the amount of DNA in the tumor cells.

Primary therapy: The principal treatment that is intended to remove cancer from the body.

Proof-of-principle: Experiment showing that a clinical theory has some physical relevance.

Prostascint scan: A radiographic body scan that uses radioactive chemicals injected into the blood stream to help locate tumor sites.

Prostate: A gland of the male reproductive system that supplies seminal fluid.

Prostatectomy: Surgical removal of the prostate gland.

Prostate specific antigen (PSA): A substance produced in minute amounts by the prostate and emitted into the blood stream. Abnormally high levels of PSA in the blood may signify disturbances of the prostate gland.

Prostatitis: Inflammation or infection of the prostate. Noncancerous.

Protocol: A defined plan for a clinical trial or medical procedure.

Proton: Sub-atomic particle often used to treat cancer.

PSA: See prostate specific antigen.

PSA density: PSA level divided by the volume of the prostate. Used in clinical predictions for cancer of the prostate.

PSA velocity: The rate of change of your PSA level over time. Used in clinical predictions for cancer of the prostate.

Radiation: High energy waves, such as X-rays, or particles, such as protons.

Radiation therapy: Use of high energy radiation to penetrate the body or a tumor to treat disease. Types of radiation may include X-rays, proton beams, electron beams, gamma rays, or alpha and beta particles.

Radical prostatectomy: Complete surgical removal of the prostate gland.

Radiologist: Physician who specializes in diagnosis or treatment utilizing radiation procedures.

Recurrence: Return of cancerous cells after primary treatment has taken place.

Refractory: Tumor cells that no longer respond to treatment control, such as becoming refractory to hormonal medicines.

Remission: When the symptoms of disease go away. Remission can be temporary or permanent.

Retropubic prostatectomy: Surgical removal of the prostate through an incision made in the lower abdomen.

Salvage surgery: Surgical treatment following primary radiation or brachytherapy therapy.

Score: As in Gleason score.

Secondary therapy: Treatment that is not expected to be the main method of cancer removal, but is hoped to augment the primary therapy.

Seminal vesicles: Glands alongside the prostate that release fluid into the semen during orgasm.

Side effect: Undesirable health conditions that are a result of treatment.

Sonogram: Ultrasound wave image of your pelvic area. Transrectal ultrasound (TRUS) technique.

Stage: The size and extent of a tumor. Can be clinical, meaning it is estimated without extensive invasive measures, or pathological as determined after removal of the prostate and surrounding tissue.

Testes: Glands in the scrotum that produce testosterone, sperm, and fluids for semen.

Testosterone: Principal male sex hormone.

Tetraploid: An aggressive tumor cell that has four times the normal number of chromosomes.

TNM staging system: System used to estimate the extent of a cancer. T stands for tumor extent, N stands for extent of lymph node involvement, and M stands for whether distant metastases are present.

Transrectal ultrasonography (TRUS): Use of sound waves to produce images of the prostate.

Transurethral resection of the prostate (TURP): Surgical removal of prostate material via the urethra. Common treatment for BPH.
Tumor: Abnormal mass or growth of tissue. Can be benign or malignant.
Urologist: Physician who specializes in diseases of the urinary tract and the reproductive system.
Whitmore-Jewett staging system: Classification system to estimate tumor stage. Categories A,B,C, and D correlate to T1,T2,T3,and T4 numbers of the TNM system.
X-ray: High energy radiation that at low levels can be used for diagnosis, and at high levels used for treatment of cancerous growths.

Appendix B

Organizations and Information Sources

These organizations operate on a nationwide level and serve as a good first stop for your investigations. This listing includes sites from which to obtain medical information as well as support group sites.

American College of Radiology
1891 Preston White Dr.
Reston, VA 22091
(800) 227-5463
www.acr.org/

American Cancer Society
1599 Clifton Road, NE
Atlanta, GA 30329
(800) 227-2345
http://www.cancer.org/

American Foundation for Urologic Disease
Prostate Cancer Support Network
Suite 401
300 West Pratt Street
Baltimore, MD 21201-2463
(800) 242-2383
http://www.afud.org

American Urological Association
1120 North Charles Street
Baltimore, MD 21201-5559
(410) 223-4310
http://www.avanet.org

Canadian Cancer Society
Suite 200
10 Alcorn Ave.
Toronto, Ontario

Canada M4V 3B1
(416) 961-7223
http://www.bc.cancer.ca/ccs/

Cancer Care, Inc.
1180 Avenue of the Americas
New York, NY 10036
(800) 813-4673
(212) 221-3300
www.cancercare.org

Cancer Hot Line
R.A. Block Cancer Foundation, Inc.
4410 Main Street
Kansas City, MO 64111
(816) 932-2853
www.cancernews.com/blockquote.html

Cancer Support Network
5895 Devereau Lane
Pittsburgh, PA 15232
(412) 661-8949
www.cancernews.com/support.html

CaP CURE
Suite 360
1250 Fourth Street
Santa Monica, CA 90401
(310) 458-2873
http://www.capcure.org

Man to Man
c/o American Cancer Society
1599 Clifton Road, NE
Atlanta, GA 30329
(800) 227-2345
www.cancer.org

National Cancer Institute (NCI)
Cancer Information Service
Room 10A24
National Institutes of Health Building 31
Bethesda, MD 20892
(800) 422-6237
wwwici.nci.nih.gov/

National Coalition for Cancer Survivorship (NCCS)
5th Floor
1010 Wayne Ave.
Silver Spring, MD 20910
(301) 650-8868
www.cansearch.org

National Institutes of Health
Patient Referral Service
Room IC 255
Building 10
9000 Rockville Pike
Bethesda, MD (301) 496-4891
www.nih.gov/

Patient Advocates for Advanced
Cancer Treatments (PAACT)
1143 Parmelee, NW
Grand Rapids, MI 49504
(616) 453-1477
http://www.osz.com/paact

US-TOO International, Inc.
Suite 50
930 North York Road
Hinsdale, IL 60521-2993
(800) 808-7866
http://www.ustoo.com

Some Internet Information Sites

American Cancer Society
http://www.cancer.org

Cancer Link
www.personal.u-net.com/~njh/cancer.html

Cancer Patient Resources
www.charm.net/~kkdk/

Cancer Treatment Centers of America
www.cancercenter.com

Cancerweb
www.graylab.ac.uk/cancerweb.html

CaP CURE
http://www.secapl.com/prostate/capcure.html

General Interest Cancer Sites
www.cancernews.com/sites.html

Doctor C.E. Koop
www.drkoop.com

National Cancer Institute
www.cancernet.nci.nih.gov
www.cancertrials.nci.nih.gov

Oncolink
http://cancer.med.upenn.edu/disease/prostate/index.html

Prostate Cancer InfoLink
http://www./comed.com/Prostate/

Prostate Pointers
www.rattler.cameron.edu/prostate/

University of Michigan Prostate Cancer Home Page
http://www.cancer.med.umich.edu/prostcan/prostcan.html

Wellness Web
http://wellweb.com/PROSTATE/prostate.html

Appendix C

Subscription Newsletters on Prostate Cancer

There are a number of subscription letters that you can obtain for relatively inexpensive fees. I list those that have been particularly helpful to me

Coping Magazine
Quarterly magazine of cancer issues and support.
P.O. Box 682268
Franklin, TN 37068-2268
(615) 790-2400

Man to Man News
Published quarterly by the American Cancer Society, this newsletter presents timely articles, new research, and notice of meetings. This letter is free.

Order this letter and obtain relevant information about American Cancer Society publications by calling them at (800) ACS-2345. Check them out at www.cancer.org.

PAACT, Inc.
The Patient Advocates for Advanced Cancer Treatments is an important support group organized throughout the United States. They publish a quarterly newsletter filled with new information. They also publish a number of information memoranda and circulate questionnaires regarding patient care, etc.

PAACT, Inc.
1143 Parmelee,
N.W. Grand Rapids, Michigan 45504-3844
(616) 453-1477
$50 contribution

Prostate Cancer Exchange

A bi-monthly letter of about two dozen pages. This is the letter published by the Education Center of Prostate Cancer Patients (ECPCP), headed up by Dr. James Lewis. Several books by Dr. Lewis are listed in the bibliography. I regard this as a must subscription.

Prostate Cancer Exchange
The Education Center for Prostate Cancer Patients
POBox 948
Westbury, New York 11590
(516) 997-1777
$30 per year

Prostate Forum

A monthly letter of a dozen or more pages packed with interesting essays. You may obtain back issues. Each month these are listed in the back of the letter.

Prostate Forum
Rivanna Health Publications
POBox 6696
Charlottesville, Virginia 22906-6696
(804) 974-1303
$36 per year

PCR Insights

A Prostate Cancer Research Institute newsletter covering many new aspects of prostate cancer treatments. The letter is free.

Prostate Cancer Research Institute
Suite 103
4676 Admiralty Way
Marina del Rey, California 90292

Appendix D

Charitable Organizations

Many organizations will receive charitable donations if you wish to contribute to efforts for research, education, and ultimately the defeat of this medical condition. Most university medical centers engage in a number of research and clinical trial programs, and would welcome any contribution you may wish to make.

American Cancer Society
1599 Clifton Road NE
Atlanta, GA 30329-4251
www.cancer.org/

Cancer Care, Inc.
1180 Avenue of the Americas
New York, NY 10036
(800) 813-4673
www.cancercareinc.org

CaP CURE
Suite 360
1250 Fourth Street
Santa Monica, CA 90401
www.capcure.org

City of Hope
1500 East Duarte Road
Duarte, CA 91010-3000
www.cityofhope.org

National Cancer Institute
Room 10A16, Building 31
31 Center Drive MSC2580
9000 Rockville Pike
Bethesda, MD 20982-2580
http://rex.nci.gov

US-TOO International, Inc.
Suite 50
930 North York Road
Hinsdale, IL 60521-2993
www.ustoo.com

Appendix E

Questions to Ask Your Physician

Talking with your doctor about cancer can be a very difficult matter for many men. But you have a right and a need to engage in frank discussions on any and all matters that will determine your future health. You are the consumer and if your physician is not fully open with you, you need to force the issue or find a physician with whom you are completely comfortable.

You are well-advised to order the National Coalition for Cancer Survivors book *Teamwork: The Cancer Patient's Guide to Talking with Your Doctor,* $2.00. NCCS, Suite 505, 1010 Wayne Ave, Silver Spring, Maryland, 20910.

Earlier I recommended that you maintain a written list of questions for your physician. I do this because it seems that whenever I enter my doctor's office my mind goes blank and I lose the train of all the ideas and thoughts that have popped into my head since the last visit. I am sure that my physicians cringe a bit when they see me coming now with my lists. Do not let this possibility deter you. And write down the responses from your physician. I know full well how short-circuited a mind can become under such emotional stress. Be sure you understand completely what your physician tells you. To do this well, you may have to be more assertive than usual. Most of all be an active listener, and do not be afraid to express your feelings. Your physicians must know how you feel, as well as how you think on what he tells you. I list a few questions that you might use to get started with your personal question list.

Annual physical exams:
If you do not have cancer there are a number of things you will want to be clear on. Some questions might be:

*Does my DRE seem normal for my age to you?

*How important is regular PSA testing to you?

*Do you utilize a local lab for PSA blood analysis or do you send it to a lab that specializes in this analysis?

*If my PSA is elevated for my age, do you obtain a free-PSA value for comparison with the bound-PSA value?

*If PSA is elevated and I have no other symptoms, do you recommend a cystoscopy or needle biopsy?

*Are you aware of the testing labs that use ultra-sensitive PSA techniques? How do we know that the PSA elevation is not merely BPH?

*If I have any prostate abnormalities according to your DRE do you recommend sonogram-guided biopsies?

*If so, how long will the procedure take? Will it hurt in any way? What medications are required in this procedure?

*Do you have diet recommendations that might lessen cancer risks?

After diagnosis for prostate cancer:
If cancer has been found there are a number of very important issues you must discuss with your physicians:

*How quickly must I decide upon a treatment option?

*What are the main issues that are important to me?

*Are you and the physicians that will be recommended to me "board certified?" Who will be involved with my care? How long have you/they been practicing medicine?

*Do you recommend a second opinion from an

oncologist, specializing in prostate cancer? If you do not recommend that I see one, why?

*Can you arrange for me to talk with a patient treated for this type of cancer?

*What is my biopsy result for Gleason type and Gleason score? Explain what these really mean to me.

*Does the biopsy show any ploidy anomalies?

*Do I need to be treated at all? What will my quality-of-life be after treatment of some kind?

*Is the tumor confined to the prostate or is there a chance that it has escaped the capsule wall? How can we be sure? Is it fast-growing or slow-growing?

*What stage is my tumor? What does this mean to me?

*Do I need sonography, a CAT scan, or a high resolution MRI to define the extent of my tumor? What will such tests tell us about my tumor?

*Please review the risks and treatment options for combating my tumor.

*What are the side effects, especially impotence and incontinence of each of these treatments?

*What are the expected benefits to me of each treatment?

*While I am investigating my treatment options should I be placed on combined hormonal medications? If so, should I not obtain a complete MRI before I begin taking hormone medication, just to establish a baseline?

*What are the chances of a recurrence of my tumor, depending upon which treatment I choose?

*If I choose surgery where should it be done? If not a

major medical center, how do the various statistics compare if done by a local doctor in a local hospital? What is the record of the surgeon for cases like mine? How many patients has he treated in the past two years?

*How long will it take to recuperate?

*How much pain will I endure? How can this be controlled?

*If I choose radiation of some kind what will it accomplish?

*How will radiation be given? How long will it take? Will I be able to continue with my normal activities? Will it be painful?

*Is the radiologist a specialist in treating patients like me? How many patients has he treated in the past two years?

*How will we know if it is successful?

*Am I a candidate for cryosurgery? If so where and by whom?

*Do you recommend any special diet or vitamin regime for me?

*What is the nearest support group that I should join?

*Are there clinical trials to investigate that are appropriate for me?

*What will the future hold for me?

*What are the costs of the various treatment options?

*What else ought I be asking of you?

Clinical trials:
If you are diagnosed with advanced cancer you will wish to explore the subject of alternative medical approaches and

clinical trials. Normally there are three phases for clinical studies. A phase 1 trial is the first step in testing a new agent in a small number of people, after the agent has been studied in laboratories. Phase 2 trials focus on learning whether or not the agent is effective in treating a cancer condition. Phase 3 trials are double-blind tests involving many subjects in the test and in a control group that utilizes a placebo, or other agent. Questions to ask might be:

*Do you recommend I investigate clinical trials? If so, can you give me information where I can find appropriate ones to consider?

*Who is the sponsor of this test? Is it fully approved?

*What does this proposed clinical trial attempt to do? Has it been tested before? What side effects can I expect from this study?

*What are the hoped for benefits to me, and what are the risks to me?

*Are there competing tests being run for men with my category of cancer?

*What information does a particular test hope to obtain?

*How many people will be in the trial?

*Who will be running this trial, and how long will it run?

*Are there medical tests performed on me during the trial? If so, what kinds of tests, and how often will they take place?

*Is it safe to take such experimental medicines?

*Will I learn the results of my trial?

*Who will now be in charge of my care? Will I still see my regular doctor?

*What will it cost me to participate? Will costs be cov-

ered by my health insurance?
***What will happen to me if I do nothing?**

Appendix F

Some Major Clinical Centers in the U.S. with Treatment Specialty

The following list of clinical centers for treating prostate cancer is brief, covering only a few of the major clinics in the United States. The National Cancer Institute can provide you with a complete list of centers for your area of the country. If there is no NCI Cancer Center in your state call (800) 4-CANCER for referrals to major cancer centers in or near your state.

1999 treatment specialties are:
(A-CL)= Alternative therapy and /or clinical trials
(B)= Brachytherapy
(C)= Cryosurgery
(P)= Proton beam
(R)= Radiation
(S)= Surgery

Northeastern U.S.

Dartmouth-Hitchcock Medical Center
Norris Cotton Cancer Center
(A-CL,B,C,R,S)
One Medical Center Drive
Lebanon, NH 03756-0001
(800) 639-6918
(603) 650-5527
http://www.nccc.hitchcock.org/

Fox Chase Cancer Center
(A-CL,B,R,S)
7701 Burholme Avenue
Philadelphia, PA 19111
(215) 728-6900
www.fccc.edu/

Johns Hopkins Oncology Center
(A-CL,B,C,R,S)
601 North Caroline Street
Baltimore, MD 21287
(410) 955-8964
www.jhu.edu/

Massachusetts General Hospital
(A-CL,B,P,R,S)
100 Blossom Street
Boston, MA 02114
(617) 726-5130
www.mgh.harvard.edu

Memorial Sloan-Kettering
Cancer Center
(A-CL,B,R,S)
1275 York Avenue
New York, NY 10021
(800) 525-2225
www.mskcc.org

University of Pennsylvania Cancer Center
(A-CL,B,R,S)
6th Floor Penn Tower
3400 Spruce Street
Philadelphia, PA 19104-4283
(215)662-6334
http://oncolink.upenn.edu

University of Rochester
Cancer Center
(A-CL,B,R,S)
601 Elmwood Avenue
Rochester, NY 14642
(716) 275-4911
www.urmc.rochester.edu/strong/cancer/cancerpg.htm

University of Vermont
Vermont Regional Cancer Center
(A-CL,B,R,S)
1 South Prospect Street
Burlington, VT 05401
(802) 656-4414
www.vtmednet.org/vcc

Yale University Cancer Center
(A-CL,B,R,S)
333 Cedar Street
New Haven, CT 06520-8028
(203) 785-2000
www.info.med.yale.edu/ycc/

Southeastern U.S.

Comprehensive Cancer Center
of Wake Forest University
(A-CL,B,R,S)
Medical Center Blvd.
Winston-Salem, NC 27157-1082
(336) 716-2075
www.bgsm.edu/cancer/

Duke Cancer Center
Duke University Medical Center
(A-CL,B,R,S)
Box 3843
Durham, NC 27710
(919) 684-8437
www.canctr.mc.duke.edu/

Virginia Commonwealth University
Massey Cancer Center
Medical College of Virginia
(A-CL,B,R,S)
Box 980037

Richmond, VA 23298-0037
(804) 828-0450
views.vcu.edu/mcc/

Radiotherapy Clinics of Georgia
(B,R)
2349 Lawrenceville Highway
Decatur, GA 30033
(800) 952-7687
(404) 320-1550
www.prostrcision.com

University of Alabama
(A-CL,B,R,S)
1824 Sixth Avenue South
Birmingham, AL 35294-3300
(800) 822-0933
www.ccc.uab.edu/

University of Miami Medical School
Sylvester Cancer Center
(A-CL,B,C,R,S)
1475 NW 12th Avenue
Miami, FL 33136
(305) 243-4300
www.sylvester.org/

Midwest and South U.S.

University Hospitals of Cleveland &
Case Western Reserve University
Ireland Cancer Center
(A-CL,B,R,S)
11100 Euclid Avenue
Cleveland, OH 44106
(800) 641-2422
(216) 844-5432
www/uhhs.com/uhc/cancer/index.html

Mayo Cancer Center
(A-CL,B,R,S)
200 First Street Southwest
Rochester, MN 55905
(507) 284-4137
www.mayo.edu/cancercenter/

Ohio State University
Comprehensive Cancer Center
(A-CL,B,R,S)
Arthur G. James Cancer Hospital
300 West 10th Avenue
Columbus, OH 43210
(800) 293-5066
www-cancer.med.ohio-state.edu/

Northwestern University
Robert H. Lurie Cancer Center
(A-CL,B,R,S)
710 N. Fairbanks Court
Chicago, IL 60611-3013
(312) 908-5250
www.nums.nwu.edu/lurie/index.html

San Antonio Cancer Institute
(A-CL,B,R,S)
8122 Datapoint Dr.
San Antonio, TX 78229-3264
(210) 616-5590
www.ccc.saci.org/

University of Colorado Cancer Center
(A-CL,B,R,S)
East Pavion Cancer Center
4200 East Ninth Avenue
Denver, CO 80262
(800) 473-2288
www.uchsc.edu/chancllr/UCCC/UCCC.html

University of Chicago
Cancer Research Center
(A-CL,B,R,S)
5841 South Maryland Avenue
Chicago, IL 60637-1470
(888) 824-0200
www uccrc.bsd.uchicago.edu/

University of Michigan
(B,R,S)
1500 E. Medical Center Dr.
Ann Arbor, MI 48109-0843
(800) 865-1125
www.cancer.med.umich.edu/

University of Wisconsin
(A-CL,B,R,S)
600 Highland Avenue
Madison, WI 53792-0001
(800) 622-8922
(608) 263-8091
http://www.ucc.wisc.edu/

Vanderbilt University
Vanderbilt Cancer Center
(A-CL,B,R,S)
649 Medical Research Building H
Nashville, TN 37232-6838
www.mc.vanderbilt.edu/uvmc/centers/cancer

Western U.S.

City of Hope National
Medical Center
(A-CL,B,R,S)
Beckman Research Institute
1500 East Duarte Road

Duarte, CA 91010
(800) 826-4673
www.cityofhope.org/

Loma Linda University Medical Center
Department of Radiation Medicine
(P, R,S)
11234 Anderson St.
Loma Linda, 92354
(800) -PROTONS
www.llu.edu/proton/

Stanford University
Medical Center
(A-CL,B,R,S)
300 Pasteur Drive
Stanford, CA 94305
(650) 723-4000
www.stanford.edu

Swedish Medical Center
Seattle Prostate Institute
(A-CL,B,R,S)
747 Broadway
Seattle, WA 98122
(206) 215-2480
www.swedish.org

University of Arizona
Arizona Cancer Center
(A-CL,B,R,S)
1515 North Campbell Avenue
Tucson, AZ 85724
(800) 622-2673
www.azcc.arizona.edu

University of California,
Davis Medical Center
(A-CL,B,R,S)
4501 X Street
Sacramento, CA 95817
(916) 734-5800
www.ucdmc.ucdavis.com/

University of California
at Irvine Cancer Center
(B,R,S)
Building 23, Route 81
101 The City Drive
Orange, CA 92668
(714) 456-8200
www.ucihealth.com/

University of California
Jonsson Comprehensive
Cancer Center
(A-CL,B,C,R,S)
10833 Le Conte Avenue
Los Angeles, CA 90095-1781
(800) 825-2631
www.cancer.mednet.ucla.edu

University of California
at San Diego Cancer Center
(A-CL,B,C,R,S)
9500 Gillman Drive
La Jolla, CA 92093-0658
(619) 543-3456
www.ucsd.edu

University of California at San Francisco (A-CL,B,C,R,S)
Long Hospital
505 Parnassus
San Francisco, CA 94143
(415) 476-4811
www.cc.ucsf.edu/

University of Hawaii at Manoa Cancer Research Center of Hawaii (A-CL, only
1236 Lauhala Street
Honolulu, HI 96813
(808) 586-3010
www2.hawaii.edu/crch

University of Utah Huntsman Cancer Institute (A-CL,B,R,S)
50 North Medical Center Drive
Salt Lake, UT 84132-5330
(800) 488-2422
www.hci.utah.edu/

University of Washington Medical Center (A-CL,B,R,S)
1959 NE Pacific Street
Seattle, WA 98195
(206) 598-4294
http://weber.u.washington.edu/~uroweb/

USC/Norris Comprehensive
Cancer Center
(A-CL,R,S)
1441 East Lake Avenue
Los Angeles, CA 90033
(323) 865-3000
www.cent.hsc.usc.edu

Appendix G

Kegel Exercises

These exercises are easy to apply and highly recommended. They will strengthen your pelvic muscles. Learn them prior to treatment and plan on utilizing them daily for the rest of our life. If you can develop this simple behavioral technique you will retain urinary control.

By flexing and relaxing these muscles you will build up tone and stamina. These exercises are remarkably effective and will cost you nothing but the time needed to make the habit automatic. Although the recommended posture is to do them while standing, I also do sitting at my desk, and while driving as well.

The standard routine Kegel exercise as developed by Beth Israel Hospital in Boston is as follows:

*While standing, squeeze the pelvic muscles, as if to hold your urine, and hold that squeeze for ten seconds. Breathe while squeezing.
*Relax for a ten second period.
*Repeat this as often as you can, perhaps ten to fifteen times, or until you are tired or unable to continue.
*Relax for a few minutes.
*Repeat with a short-cycle exercise: Squeeze for one or two seconds, relax for a second or two. Repeat a dozen times, then rest for a few moments.
*Repeat this short-cycle exercise ten times.
*Do these exercises as often as your physician suggests.

About the Author

Will Connell was born in 1935 and raised in Los Angeles. After attending the University of California at Berkeley and receiving a degree in mining geology he obtained a commission with the United States Coast and Geodetic Survey. While with the Survey he spent almost three years engaged in oceanographic and hydrographic work at sea.

After graduate work at Berkeley and at the University of Southern California, where he studied astro-geology, he spent fifteen years working in the aerospace engineering field. Work here included experiments on the X-15 rocket plane, and with our manned lunar missions.

He has two grown children, each following professional careers.

Since 1990 he has lived in Grass Valley, California, where he pursues his interest in sculpture. He expects to continue doing so for the next thirty years at least!

Two months after being diagnosed with prostate cancer and six months prior to treatment, he was married. This event was testimony to love and caring, and to a full and fulfilling future.

Publications

1996 "Beyond Buyer Beware": *In Evaluating and Implementing Hedge Fund Strategies.* Euromoney Books.

1970 *Contrast Improvement in Display Systems.* McDonnell Douglas.

1966 *Remote Multispectral Sensing of the Earth.* McDonnell Douglas. Used as textbook at UC.

Index

Order Form

Prostate Cancer Treatment Options
A Guide to the Basics

Name:______________________________________
Address:____________________________________
City:__________**State:**__________**Zip:** _____________

Postal orders:
Edconco Press
PO Box 357
Grass Valley
California
95945

Internet Site:
www.prostatecanceroptions.com

_______copies at $19.95 each = ..._____
Shipping and handling $1.75 per book = ..._____
Shipping and handling outside U.S. $2.50 = . . ._____
California residents add $1.55 sales tax per book = _____
Total = ..._____

Please send information on upcoming books and guides on medical issues:
Yes____No____

Order Form

Prostate Cancer Treatment Options
A Guide to the Basics

Name:______________________________________
Address:____________________________________
City:__________**State:**__________**Zip:** _____________

Postal orders:
Edconco Press
PO Box 357
Grass Valley
California
94945

Internet Site:
www.prostatecanceroptions.com

_______copies at $19.95 each = ..._____
Shipping and handling $1.75 per book = ..._____
Shipping and handling outside U.S. $2.50 = . . ._____
California residents add $1.55 sales tax per book = _____
Total = ..._____

Please send information on upcoming books and guides on medical issues:
Yes____No____